PocketRadiologist™
Chest
Top 100 Diagnoses

PocketRadiologist™
Chest
Top 100 Diagnoses

Jud W Gurney MD FACR
Charles A Dobry Professor of Radiology
University of Nebraska Medical Center
Omaha, Nebraska

Helen T Winer-Muram MD
Professor of Radiology
Indiana University Medical Center
Indianapolis, Indiana

With 200 drawings and radiographic images

Drawings: *Lane R Bennion MS*
                    Richard Coombs MS
                    James A Cooper MD
                    Walter Stuart MFA

Image Editing: *Ming Q Huang MD*
                    Danielle Morris
                    Melissa Petersen

Medical Text Editing: *Richard H Wiggins III MD*

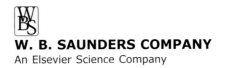

W. B. SAUNDERS COMPANY
An Elsevier Science Company

AMIRSYS™

A medical reference publishing company

First Edition

Text - Copyright Jud W Gurney MD FACR 2003

Drawings - Copyright Amirsys Inc 2003

Compilation - Copyright Amirsys Inc 2003

First Printing: November 2002

Composition by Amirsys Inc, Salt Lake City, Utah

Printed by K/P Corporation, Salt Lake City, Utah

ISBN: 0-7216-9704-6

Preface

The **PocketRadiologist™** series is an innovative, quick reference designed to deliver succinct, up-to-date information to practicing professionals "at the point of service." As close as your pocket, each title in the series is written by world-renowned authors. These experts have designated the "top 100" diagnoses or interventional procedures in every major body area, bulleted the most essential facts, and offered high-resolution imaging to illustrate each topic. Selected references are included for further review. Full color anatomic-pathologic computer graphics model many of the actual diseases.

Each **PocketRadiologist™** title follows an identical format. The same information is in the same place - every time - and takes you quickly from key facts to imaging findings, differential diagnosis, pathology, pathophysiology, and relevant clinical information. The interventional modules give you the essentials and "how-tos" of important procedures, including pre- and post-procedure checklists, common problems and complications.

PocketRadiologist™ titles are available in both print and hand-held PDA formats. Currently available modules feature Brain, Head and Neck, Orthopedic (Musculoskeletal) Imaging, Pediatrics, Spine, Chest, Cardiac, Vascular, Abdominal Imaging and Interventional Radiology. 2003 topics will include Obstetrics, Gynecologic Imaging, Breast, and much, much more. Enjoy!

Anne G Osborn MD
Editor-in-Chief, Amirsys Inc

H Ric Harnsberger
Chairman and CEO, Amirsys Inc

Notice and Disclaimer

PocketRadiologist™
Chest
Top 100 Diagnoses

The diagnoses in this book are divided into 14 sections in the following order:

Airspace
Airways
Interstitial
Mediastinum
Carcinoma
Nodule(s)
Pleura
Hyperinflation & Cysts
Heart & Pericardial
Pulmonary Artery
Aorta
Trauma
Portable ICU
Chest Wall

Table of Contents

Airspace

Airways

Interstitial

Table of Contents

Mediastinum

Carcinoma

Nodule(s)

Table of Contents

PocketRadiologist™
Chest
Top 100 Diagnoses

AIRSPACE

Diffuse Alveolar Damage

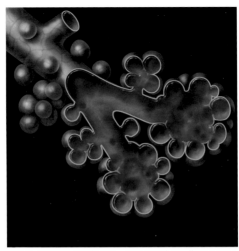

Adult respiratory distress syndrome. Increased capillary permeability with proteinaceous hemorrhagic fluid filling alveoli. Other features include hyaline membrane formation, alveolar atelectasis and small vessel microthomboses.

Key Facts
- Diffuse peripheral pulmonary consolidation
- Lack of Kerley B lines and peribronchial cuffing
- Anterior (nondependent) cysts from barotrauma with positive end-expiratory pressure (PEEP)
- Acute respiratory distress syndrome (ARDS): Clinical definition, severe hypoxemia on high concentrations of O_2, normal wedge pressure
- Seen with nearly any medical or surgical condition: Toxic fumes, aspiration, shock, postoperative, pancreatitis

Imaging Findings
General Features
- Best imaging clue: Intubated patient with diffuse peripheral consolidation
Chest Radiograph
- Diffuse pulmonary consolidation
- Favors the lung periphery
- Kerley B lines infrequent (more frequent with cardiogenic edema)
- Peribronchial cuffing infrequent
- Normal heart size: No pulmonary vascular redistribution
- May have small pleural effusions
- Initial use of PEEP may increase lung volume giving apparent radiographic "improvement"
- Barotrauma common with PEEP
- Superimposed pneumonia common
CT/HRCT Findings
- Surprisingly inhomogeneous
- Gravitational gradient: Ventral to dorsal increase in opacities
- PEEP may overdistend less involved ventral lung, leads to cysts & bullae
- Resolution, coarse reticular thickening and cyst formation in anterior (ventral, nondependent) lung

Diffuse Alveolar Damage

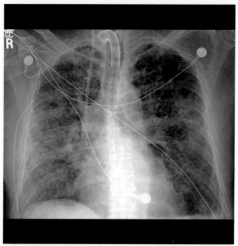

Diffuse interstitial thickening and consolidation. Long term tracheostomy. Cystic lucencies in the left mid lung and left upper lobe may represent ventral cysts from barotrauma.

Imaging Recommendations
- Chest radiography
  - To evaluate extent of parenchymal disease
  - Location of support and monitoring apparatus
  - To detect complications of barotrauma
- CT
  - For complications of barotrauma, i.e., pneumatocele, pneumothorax, pneumomediastinum
  - For complications of infection, i.e., lung abscess, empyema

Differential Diagnosis
General
- Usually patients with ARDS rapidly intubated to support oxygenation even when severity of consolidation mild
- Rather than radiographic differentiation, clinical management based on Swan-Ganz catheter and pulmonary capillary wedge pressure (PCWP)
Cardiogenic Edema
- Separation from cardiogenic pulmonary edema moderately successful
  - Absent Kerley B lines and peribronchial cuffing
  - Peripheral predominance
  - Normal heart size, pleural effusions rare
  - No pulmonary vascular redistribution, normal vascular pedicle
Pneumonia
- May have identical radiographic findings, may result in ARDS
Massive Aspiration
- May have identical radiographic findings, may result in ARDS
Hemorrhage
- May have identical radiographic findings, patient often anemic

Diffuse Alveolar Damage

Pathology

General
- Good correlation between radiographic patterns and pathologic changes
- Common misconception that insult is homogeneous
- 3 phases
  - Exudative phase: Normal at HRCT
  - Proliferative phase: Ground-glass opacities to frank consolidation
    - Even though capillary injury is diffuse, lung opacities most severe in the dependent lung from fluid accumulation and atelectasis
  - Chronic phase: Resolution of consolidation, residual scarring and cysts
    - Cyst formation and coarse reticular thickening, particularly in nondependent lung due to PEEP barotrauma
- Pathophysiology: Inflammatory mediators damage capillary membrane
- Etiology
  - Nearly any major medical or surgical condition
    - Airway insult; aspiration (especially gastric acid); toxic fume inhalation; O_2 toxicity; pneumonia
    - Blood-borne insult; sepsis; transfusion; surgery; shock; eclampsia; pancreatitis

Gross Pathologic Features
- Exudative: Heavy, airless, deep purple lung
- Hepatization of lung fibrosis, cysts: May eventually return to normal

Microscopic Features
- Diffuse alveolar damage (DAD)
  - Exudative: Capillary congestion, microatelectasis
  - Proliferative: Protein-rich interstitial edema, hyaline membranes
  - Chronic: Hyperplasia type II pneumocyte, fibroblastic infiltration

Staging or Grading Criteria
- Stage 1: Exudative (first 24 hours)
- Stage 2: Proliferative (1-7 days)
- Stage 3: Chronic (>1 week)

Clinical Issues

Presentation
- Acute (immediate) or insidious (hours or days) after initiating event
- Dyspnea, tachypnea, dry cough, agitation, cyanosis
- ARDS clinical definition for DAD, $P_aO_2 < 50$ with $F_iO_2 > 50\%$
- Normal wedge pressure: Decreased lung compliance
- May have no chest radiographic abnormalities in first 12 hours
- Later, chest radiograph diffusely abnormal

Treatment
- Steroids or extracorporeal membrane oxygenation (ECMO) not shown to be beneficial; supportive, mechanical ventilation: PEEP

Prognosis
- High mortality rate
- Survivors may have either restrictive or obstructive functional deficits

Selected References
1. Goodman LR et al: Congestive heart failure and adult respiratory distress syndrome. New insights using computed tomography. Radiol Clin North Am 34: 33-46, 1996
2. Maunder RJ et al: Preservation of normal lung regions in the adult respiratory distress syndrome. Analysis by computed tomography. JAMA 255:2463-5, 1986
3. Ashbaugh DG et al: Acute respiratory distress in adults. Lancet 2:319-23, 1967

Aspiration Pneumonia

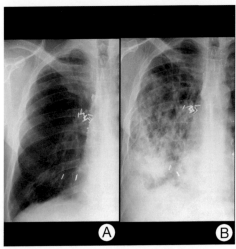

Previous right upper lobectomy. Coughing up metallic clips, recurrent pneumonia due to clip aspiration. Note: Changed position of clips between (A) and (B).

Key Facts
- Pulmonary inflammation due to aspiration of infected oropharyngeal secretions
- Patients may be unconscious, post-operation, intubated or have gastro-esophageal disorders
- Gravity-dependent opacities, usually bilateral, basal and perihilar
- Recurrent pneumonias in chronic aspiration
- Aspiration of gastric acid during labor and delivery can be severe and fatal (Mendelson's syndrome)

Imaging Findings
General Features
- Best imaging clue: Recurrent gravity-dependent opacities

Chest Radiograph
- Acute aspiration
  - Gravity-dependent, patchy, multi-focal airspace opacities, usually bilateral (conversely may be unilateral), basal and perihilar
  - Supine position; posterior segments of upper lobes or superior segments of lower lobes
  - Airway findings from larger aspirated particles
    - Segmental or lobar atelectasis
    - Hyperinflation or air trapping more common in infants and children
  - May worsen in first few days then clear rapidly
  - Aspiration of large amounts of gastric contents can progress to acute respiratory distress syndrome (ARDS) (Mendelson's syndrome)
  - Complications: Necrotizing pneumonia, abscess, ARDS, pulmonary embolism
- Chronic aspiration
  - Recurrent opacities often in the same location, reticulonodular opacities, bronchiectasis, pulmonary fibrosis

Aspiration Pneumonia

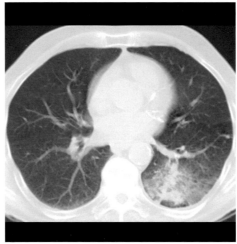

Aspiration pneumonia. CT lower lobe. Consolidation and ground-glass opacities in the superior segment of the left lower lobe. History of recurrent bilateral pneumonias and gastroesophageal reflux. Differential with this history includes lipoid pneumonia, and drowned lung.

CT Findings
- Airspace opacities in dependent lung, centrilobular nodules
- Can be used to evaluate for complications of abscess, empyema

Imaging Recommendations
- In infants, decubitus films to investigate air trapping
- Scintigraphy with radio-labeled food to document aspiration

Differential Diagnosis

Pneumonia or Recurrent Pneumonias
- Identical radiographic findings
- Immunocompromised patient predisposed to recurrent pneumonias

Pulmonary Embolism
- Identical radiographic findings
- Infarcts peripheral, often with pleural effusion
- Predisposing factors for thromboembolism

Pulmonary Edema
- Cardiomegaly, pleural effusions
- Kerley B lines uncommon with aspiration

ARDS
- Identical radiographic findings
- Aspiration predisposing factor for ARDS

Bronchiolitis Obliterans Organizing Pneumonia (BOOP)
- Similar radiographic findings, may also wax and wane

Pathology

General
- Etiology-pathogenesis-pathophysiology
  - Amount of pulmonary damage depends on amount and nature of aspirated material

Aspiration Pneumonia

- o Aspiration of gastric acid during labor and delivery can be severe and fatal (Mendelson's syndrome)
- Epidemiology
  - o Not uncommon, may be subclinical and chronic
  - o Most common in healthy infants and small children
  - o Adults often have underlying conditions, e.g., neurologic disorders, alcoholism, esophageal disorders, on mechanical ventilation, tracheoesophageal fistula
  - o Can occur in healthy adults while eating solid food (café coronary)

Gross Pathologic-Surgical Features
- Food particles or teeth may be noted within the airways
- Edema and acute inflammation of airway (acutely)
- Air-space edema, hemorrhage, organizing bronchopneumonia, bacterial abscesses (acutely): Bronchiectasis and fibrosis (chronically)

Microscopic Features
- Airway
  - o Incorporation of foreign material in granulation tissue
  - o Intraluminal granulation tissue, bronchostenosis, or bronchiectasis
- Lung
  - o Neutrophils, mononuclear cells and giant cells, < 48 hours
  - o Pneumonia often due to aerobic, anaerobic, or actinomycosis infection
  - o In chronic disease, features include recurrent pneumonia, well-organized granulomas, obliterative bronchiolitis, bronchiectasis, and fibrosis

Clinical Issues
Presentation
- Acute onset with choking, cough, cyanosis, hypoxemia, loss of consciousness
- Insidious onset, with repeated aspiration and recurrent pneumonias
- May resemble asthma or acute myocardial infarction
- Predisposition: Debilitated, unconscious patients, alcoholism, intubation or nasogastric tubes in place or patients with disorders affecting swallowing, i.e., gastroesophageal reflux, Zenker's diverticulum, esophageal stricture

Treatment
- Bronchoscopy to remove foreign bodies, i.e., peanuts, beans, teeth, etc.
- Antibiotics, medications to reduce gastric pH, gastric suction with nasogastric tube
- Elevation of head, surgery for chronic gastroesophageal reflux

Prognosis
- Death rate for patients who develop ARDS from Mendelson's syndrome is up to 50%

Selected References
1. Franquet T et al: Aspiration diseases: Findings, pitfalls, and differential diagnosis. Radiographics 20:673-85, 2000
2. Marom EM et al: The many faces of pulmonary aspiration. AJR 172: 121-8, 1999
3. Bartlett JG et al: The triple threat of aspiration pneumonia. Chest 68:560-6, 1975

Atelectasis

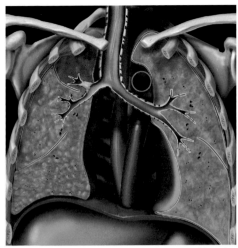

Right upper lobe atelectasis results in superior displacement of the minor fissure and right hilum, bowing of the trachea to the right and hyperaeration of the right middle and lower lobes.

Key Facts
- Decrease in volume of lung or a portion of lung
- Types: Obstructive, passive, cicatrizing, and adhesive
- Signs: Shift of fissures, mediastinum and hila toward collapse
- Diagnosis can be made with chest radiography: CT establish cause

Imaging Findings
General Features
- Best imaging clue: Displacement of fissures
- Types of atelectasis
  - Obstructive, e.g., bronchial neoplasm, no air bronchograms
  - Passive, e.g., pneumothorax or pleural effusion - lung volume loss in proportion to volume of occupied pleural space
  - Cicatrizing, e.g., remote tuberculosis with volume loss due to scarring
  - Adhesive, e.g., ARDS collapse due to surfactant deficiency
- Lobar collapse
  - Airlessness of affected lobe, local increase in opacity
  - Total lung volume average = 6720 ml
  - Signs of atelectasis proportional to amount of volume loss
  - Crowding of vessels and bronchi in affected lobe
  - Displacement of fissures, mediastinum, and hilum towards the collapse
  - Overinflation of remaining lobes
  - "Silhouette" sign – loss of air – soft tissue interface when collapsed lung abuts an adjacent soft-tissue structure

Chest Radiograph
- Right upper lobe (RUL) atelectasis (average volume RUL = 1140 ml)
  - Collapses superiorly and medially, loss of SVC interface and apical soft-tissue capping
  - PA - lateral radiograph: Minor fissure displaced upward
  - Lateral: Superior aspect of major fissure displaced anteriorly

Atelectasis

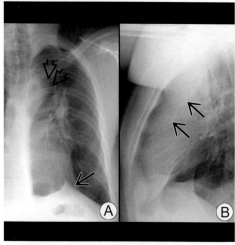

Left upper lobe atelectasis. Indirect signs frontal radiograph (A), elevation left hilum, and diaphragm and mediastinal shift. Left juxtaphrenic peak (arrows) and luftsichel (open arrows). On the lateral (B), the major fissure is displaced anteriorl (arrow).

- o Central mass: "Reverse S sign of Golden"
- o Juxtaphrenic peak: Tent of diaphragm (due to upward retraction inferior accessory fissure)
- Left upper lobe (LUL) atelectasis (average volume LUL = 1160 ml)
  - o Collapses anteriorly, partial loss of left heart border, haze superimposed on left hilum
  - o Lateral: Major fissure shifted anteriorly
  - o Luftsichel sign: Superior segment of lower lobe causes a crescent lucency between the aortic arch and the atelectatic upper lobe
- Right middle lobe (RML) atelectasis (average volume RML = 670 ml)
  - o Collapses as a triangle toward the right heart border
  - o PA: Obscuration of right heart border
  - o Lateral: Thin triangle or pancake shape from anterior chest wall with apex toward hilum, inferior displacement of minor fissure, anterior-superior displacement of inferior aspect of major fissure
- Lower lobe atelectasis (average volume LLL = 1550 ml, RLL 2000 ml)
  - o Collapses posteriorly, medially and inferiorly
  - o PA: Triangular opacity medial lung bases obscures diaphragms
  - o Lateral: Posterior displacement of major fissure, vague opacity over lower thoracic spine
- Right middle and lower lobe atelectasis
  - o Similar to pleural effusion: Ill-defined right heart border and diaphragm
  - o Pathology involving bronchus intermedius
- Right upper and right middle lobe atelectasis
  - o Simulates left upper lobe atelectasis (double bronchus sign: 2 separate airways obstructed)
  - o Borrie's sump: Nodes between RUL and RML bronchus may obstruct both
  - o Bronchogenic carcinoma most common cause

Atelectasis

- Segmental and subsegmental atelectasis (plate atelectasis)
  - Long linear opacities are thicker and more indistinct than Kerley B lines
  - Indicates low volume states; common in critically ill or post-op patients
  - Also seen with pulmonary embolism
- Total lung atelectasis
  - Shift of mediastinum to opacity, hyperinflation of contralateral lung
  - Differentiation large pleural effusion: Mediastinal shift to opposite side
- Round Atelectasis
  - Associated with pleural thickening (asbestos related) in lower lobes
  - Oval, wedge-shaped, or irregular subpleural mass with air bronchograms (60%)
  - Comet tail sign (whorled bronchovascular markings into mass)
  - Most are stable for many years

CT Findings
- Can help identify cause, i.e., bronchial obstructing lesion
- No imaging can predict if the atelectatic lobe is sterile or infected

Imaging Recommendations
- CT useful to exclude endobronchial lesion and confirm round atelectasis

Differential Diagnosis
Pneumonia
- Radiographic opacity but no volume loss

Embolus
- Peripheral opacity, volume loss of hemithorax due to splinting

Lung Cancer
- Round atelectasis may simulate lung cancer
- Endobronchial neoplasm common cause of lobar atelectasis in adult

Pathology
General
- Lobar obstruction, collapse in 18 to 24 hours if breathing room air
- Lobar obstruction, collapse in < 5 minutes if breathing 100% oxygen
  - Nitrogen very slowly absorbed, delays development of atelectasis
- Obstructed lobe may not collapse because of ventilation across the pores of Kohn and canals of Lambert, or across incomplete fissures

Microscopic Features
- No specific features, most biopsy specimens atelectatic

Clinical Issues
Presentation
- Asymptomatic, fever can occur with atelectasis without infection
- Left lower lobe collapse: Most common in ICU setting

Treatment
- Atelectasis not a disease, treatment aimed at underlying cause

Prognosis
- Determined by underlying cause

Selected References
1. Proto AV et al: Radiographic manifestations of lobar collapse. Semin Roentgenol 15: 117-73, 1980

Cryptogenic Organizing Pneumonia

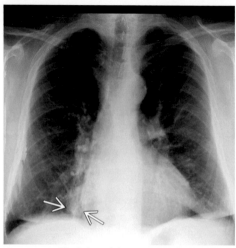

Nonspecific air-space opacities in lower lobes, most prominent on the right (arrows). No change from previous films obtained 3 months earlier.

Key Facts
- Synonym: Proliferative bronchiolitis obliterans, bronchiolitis obliterans organizing pneumonia (BOOP)
- Patchy peripheral consolidation, slight preference for lower lung zones
- Other patterns: Lobular-sized nodules, solitary mass, diffuse interstitial thickening
- Causes: Idiopathic, infection, drugs, transplants, toxic fume inhalation
- Cough, shortness of breath (SOB), low-grade fever
- Restrictive pulmonary function tests
- Steroid responsive

Imaging Findings
General Features
- Best imaging clue: Chronic peripheral, basilar, patchy consolidation
Chest Radiograph
- Patchy, bilateral, variable-sized areas of consolidation
- Unilateral 5%
- Favors the lower lung zones
- Normal heart size, no adenopathy
- Lung volumes preserved
- Less common: Solitary mass (usually upper lung zone)
- Less common: Diffuse reticular interstitial thickening
- May wax and wane (also termed migration)
CT/HRCT Findings
- Peripheral opacities range from ground-glass density to consolidation
- Consolidation often triangular in shape
- Consolidation may extend along bronchi (peribronchovascular pattern)
- Mild mediastinal adenopathy common (not seen in chest radiographs)
- Lobular-sized nodules with well-defined margins in random distribution
- Diffuse, reticular, interstitial thickening primarily basilar is less common

Cryptogenic Organizing Pneumonia

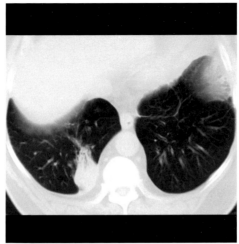

CT better defines the opacities within the lung. Peripheral basilar areas of consolidation with air bronchograms. Typical findings for BOOP or cryptogenic organizing pneumonia.

- Solitary mass may have air bronchograms or cavitate, usually upper lobe location
- Occasional small effusion

Imaging Recommendations
- Chest radiographs usually sufficient for characterization and follow-up
- CT may be useful to characterize pulmonary disease and to exclude pulmonary embolism

Differential Diagnosis
Chronic Eosinophilic Pneumonia
- Eosinophilic pneumonia usually upper lung zone (eosinophilia absent in BOOP)

Usual Interstitial Pneumonia (UIP)
- Honeycombing and decreased lung volumes (absent in BOOP)

Lymphoma
- Pulmonary lymphoma usually secondary to known disease
- Adenopathy in other lymph node groups
- No peripheral predominance, often centered on bronchi

Bronchioloalveolar Cell Carcinoma (BAC)
- BAC not predominately subpleural, BAC usually ground-glass density

Sarcoid
- No peripheral predominance
- May be associated with symmetric hilar adenopathy

Lung Cancer (Solitary Mass)
- No distinguishing features, diagnosis by fine needle biopsy

Aspiration
- Opacities not as chronic or peripheral as BOOP

Mycobacterial Infection
- Often cavitary in upper lobe location

Cryptogenic Organizing Pneumonia

- Old disease associated with volume loss and bronchiectasis (not seen with BOOP)

Lipoid Pneumonia
- Lipoid pneumonia may have fat density in areas of consolidated lung at CT

Pulmonary Embolism
- Multiple infarcts peripherally located in bases (identical to BOOP)
- Usually associated with pleural effusions
- Known risk factors for thromboembolism

Pathology
General
- Contrary to name, primary pathology located in alveolus and secondarily extends into small airways
- Etiology-Pathogenesis-Pathophysiology
  - Idiopathic
  - Infection (mycoplasma, viruses, atypical bacteria)
  - Drugs (amiodarone, bleomycin, sulfasalazine)
  - Connective tissue disease (rheumatoid arthritis, Sjögren's)
  - Transplant (lung, bone marrow)
  - Toxic fume inhalation (silo filler's disease)
  - Radiation therapy
  - Aspiration
  - Wegener's granuloma

Gross Pathologic-Surgical Features
- Lung architecture preserved (no fibrosis)
- Granulation tissue extends into airway lumen (bronchiolitis component)

Microscopic Features
- Buds of loosely organized granulation tissue extend through pores of Kohn to next alveolus ("butterfly" pattern)
- Mononuclear cell interstitial infiltration admixed with other inflammatory cells, no specific microscopic feature

Clinical Issues
Presentation
- Adults, no gender preference
- Cough
- SOB
- Low-grade fever
- Pulmonary function test usually restrictive, may be mixed restrictive and obstructive

Natural History
- Usually waxes and wanes, often treated for months for "recurrent" pneumonia

Treatment and Prognosis
- Steroids, less dramatic response than eosinophilic pneumonia
- Resolves over period of weeks
- Good, may relapse on discontinuation of steroids

Selected References
1. Cordier JF: Organising pneumonia. Thorax 55:318-28, 2000
2. Lee KS: Cryptogenic organizing pneumonia: CT findings in 43 patients. AJR 162:543-6, 1994
3. Davison AG et al: Cryptogenic organizing pneumonitis. Q J Med 52:382-94, 1983

Alveolar Cell Carcinoma

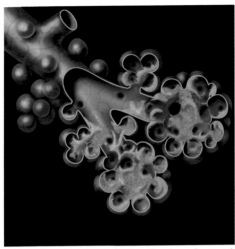

Bronchioloalveolar cell carcinoma spreads along the airway framework of the lung without invasion of interstitium. Patent small bronchioles and small cystic spaces within the tumor are often seen as air bronchiolograms.

Key Facts
- Lung cancer: Subtype of adenocarcinoma
- Small peripheral nodule most common radiographic abnormality
- Consolidation - segmental, lobar, multifocal or multilobar seen with radiography simulates pneumonia
- CT used to show extent of disease and for staging
- Synonym: Bronchioloalveolar cell carcinoma
- Best prognosis for patients with peripheral nodule
- Poorest prognosis in patients with diffuse disease and bronchorrhea

Imaging Findings
General Features
- Best imaging clue: Chronic multilobar consolidation
Chest Radiograph
- Solitary or multiple peripheral nodules
- Focal or multiple, ill-defined, hazy opacities
- Airspace opacification – localized or widespread, with air bronchograms
- Simulates pneumonia
- Lobar atelectasis without air bronchogram: Rare
- Elongated opacity simulating mucoid impaction: Rare
CT Findings
- May show additional areas of involvement, lung, pleura, mediastinum
- Nodule(s), often subpleural with pleural retraction and a central scar
- Nodules may have bubble-like lucencies
- Ground-glass opacification, focal or multifocal
- Dense consolidation with air bronchograms, focal or multifocal
- Lobar consolidation with volume loss or increased volume
- CT angiogram sign: Contrast-enhanced vessels through low attenuation consolidation
- Calcification from psammoma bodies (rare)

Alveolar Cell Carcinoma

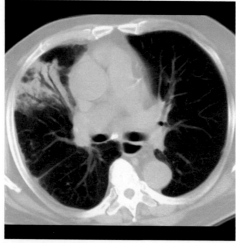

Bronchioloalveolar cell carcinoma. Nonspecific consolidation throughout the right middle lobe. Differential for chronic consolidation would include aspiration, lymphoma, pseudolymphoma, and chronic pneumonia.

Imaging Recommendations
- CT useful to investigate chronic consolidation, nodular ground-glass opacities highly suspicious for bronchioloalveolar carcinoma (BAC)
- Often no uptake with PET imaging

Differential Diagnosis
Pneumonia
- Will respond and regress with appropriate antibiotics (BAC will not improve with antibiotics)
Hemorrhage
- Will slowly resolve over 10-14 days (not seen with BAC)
Edema
- Will respond to diuretics
- Tends not to have ground-glass nodular pattern
- Kerley B lines uncommon with BAC
Aspiration
- Gravity-dependent location
- Resolves, time dependent on quality of aspirate
Bronchiolitis Obliterans Organizing Pneumonia (BOOP)
- Peripheral nodular consolidation
- Tends to wax and wane (not seen with BAC)
- Responds to steroid treatment (no effect with BAC)

Pathology
General
- Subtype of adenocarcinoma
- May arise from bronchiolar and alveolar epithelium, Clara cells
- Lipidic growth: Tumor cells spread using the underlying pulmonary architecture as scaffolding without distortion of the surrounding lung
- Etiology-Pathogenesis-Pathophysiology

Alveolar Cell Carcinoma

o Bronchogenic spread: Tumor cells may spread to other lobes or contralateral lung via the tracheobronchial tree
o May arise from bronchogenic cyst or congenital cystic adenomatoid malformation

Gross Pathologic-Surgical Features
• Mucinous and non-mucinous forms

Microscopic Features
• Malignant cells lining the alveoli and small airways (lipidic growth)

Staging
• TNM classification, as with other pulmonary carcinomas

Clinical Issues

Presentation
• Age > 40
• Peripheral nodules usually found incidentally with chest radiography
• With mucinous type: Cough and bronchorrhea may be severe
• Diagnosis by sputum cytology, fine needle aspiration biopsy or transbronchial biopsy

Treatment
• Surgical resection for localized disease
• Radiation therapy and chemotherapy for disseminated disease

Prognosis
• Peripheral nodule: When resected, 75% 5-year survival
• Despite 5 year "cure" may recur up to 20 years later
• Worse prognosis with diffuse form of disease
• Poorer prognosis with mucinous tumors than with nonmucinous tumors

Selected References
1. Lee KS et al: Bronchioloalveolar carcinoma: Clinical, histopathologic, and radiologic findings. Radiographics 17:1345-57, 1997
2. Jang HJ et al: Bronchioloalveolar carcinoma: Focal area of ground-glass attenuation at thin-section CT as an early sign. Radiology 199:485-8, 1996
3. Adler B et al: High-resolution CT of bronchioloalveolar carcinoma. AJR 159:275-7, 1992

Cardiogenic Pulmonary Edema

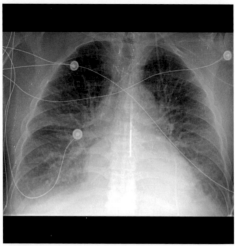

Cardiogenic pulmonary edema post myocardial infarction. Heart is mildly enlarged.
Upper lobe veins are distended (pulmonary venous hypertension). Batwing distribution
of central edema obscures vessel margins.

Key Facts
- Common problem usually due to left heart failure
- Stepwise progression from pulmonary venous hypertension to interstitial edema to alveolar edema
- Can clear rapidly with treatment
- Shifts gradually with position (gravitational shift test)

Imaging Findings
Общие Features

General Features
- Best imaging clue: Cardiomegaly with pulmonary venous hypertension and interstitial edema

Chest Radiograph
- Earliest radiographic manifestation: Upper lobe vessels are equal to or larger in diameter than lower lobe vessels; increased pulmonary artery/bronchus ratio in upper lobes, ill-defined lower lung vessels
- Interstitial edema - thickening of interlobular septa - Kerley A and B lines, lower zonal and perihilar haze, subpleural edema thickens interlobar fissures, peribronchial cuffing
    - Kerley A: Long lines in upper lobes radiating towards hilum (rare)
    - Kerley B: Short, peripheral, perpendicular lines generally in lower lobes (common)
- Alveolar edema - diffuse airspace opacification - gravity dependent
- "Bat's wing" (butterfly, perihilar) opacities (uncommon)
- Small bilateral effusions, larger on right, rarely unilateral on the left
- Cardiac enlargement chronically (normal heart with acute myocardial ischemia or arrhythmia)
- In chronic obstructive pulmonary disease (COPD), the cardiac size is often small due to hyperinflation, subsequent increases in heart size may not be beyond the range of normal
- Azygos $\pm$ SVC distention (widened vascular pedicle)

Cardiogenic Pulmonary Edema

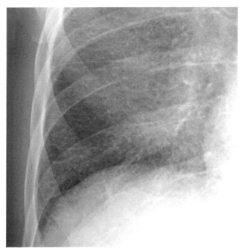

Kerley B lines. Short perpendicular lines represent edema in the walls and of lymphatics of the secondary pulmonary lobules.

- Temporal relationship of pressure and volume
  - Acute pressure (capillary wedge pressure) elevation
    - Initially normal, edema accumulates over 12-hour period
  - Pressure decrease with treatment
    - Edema resolves hours to days; radiograph "lags" clinical course

<u>CT/HRCT Findings</u>
- Chest radiograph equivalents, smooth thickening of interlobular septa, bronchovascular bundle thickening, gravity-dependent ground-glass and/or airspace opacities

<u>Imaging Recommendations</u>
- Chest radiographs sufficient for diagnosis and monitoring

Differential Diagnosis
<u>Interstitial Edema</u>
- Pneumonia
  - Febrile, usually viral or mycoplasma etiology
  - Heart normal size
  - Usually no pleural effusion
- Lymphangitic carcinomatosis
  - Normal heart size
  - Known history of malignancy
  - Usually not diffuse like pulmonary edema
  - Lymphadenopathy

<u>Alveolar Edema</u>
- Non-cardiogenic edema
  - More often acute respiratory distress syndrome (ARDS) peripheral, chronic heart failure (CHF) "bat's wing"
  - Pleural effusions unusual with ARDS
  - ARDS patients usually require intubation to support ventilation
- Pneumonia
  - Identical radiographic findings

Cardiogenic Pulmonary Edema

- o Heart usually normal in size
- o Pneumonia will not shift with gravity (gravitational shift test)
- Pulmonary hemorrhage
  - o Normal heart size with no pleural effusions
  - o Patients usually anemic
  - o Hemorrhage will not shift with gravity (gravitational shift test)
- Alveolar proteinosis
  - o "Bat's wing" pattern identical to CHF, patients asymptomatic
  - o Heart size will be normal with no pleural effusions
- Acute eosinophilic pneumonia
  - o Heart size normal with no pleural effusions
  - o Patients usually younger and have fever

Interstitial Edema, Cardiomegaly, Pleural Effusions
- Erdheim-Chester disease (rare, non-Langerhans cell granulomatosis)
  - o Will not respond to diuretics
  - o Sclerotic bone lesions

Pathology
General
- Imbalance in Starling forces
- Increase in microvascular pressure increases endothelial gaps
- Transvascular (low protein content) fluid moves into interstitial spaces
- Alveolar edema permeates across the alveolar-capillary membrane
- Lymphatic flow increases in chronic edema (10 fold), but not acute edema
- Etiology-pathogenesis
  - o Pulmonary venous hypertension (PVHTN) is usually due to left heart failure (e.g., myocardial infarction, ischemic cardiomyopathy)
  - o Other causes include mitral valve disease, left atrial myxoma, veno-occlusive disease, fibrosing mediastinitis
  - o PVHTN elevates microvascular pressure
  - o Fluid flows into interstitial spaces – rate depends on hydrostatic and osmotic pressures in vessels, interstitium, and lymphatics
  - o Upper zone vascular distention with wedge pressures of 12-18 mm Hg
  - o Kerley lines develop when wedge pressures reach 20–25 mm Hg
  - o Alveolar edema develops with wedge pressures of 25-30 mm Hg

Clinical Issues
Presentation
- Onset can be acute or insidious
- Symptoms include respiratory distress, orthopnea, anxiety
- May expectorate frothy, blood-tinged sputum
- Pulmonary function tests show decreased lung compliance
- Superimposed pulmonary embolus more likely to result in infarction

Treatment
- Oxygen, diuretics, morphine, afterload reduction and inotropic agents

Selected References
1. Gluecker T et al: Clinical and radiologic features of pulmonary edema. Radiographics 19:1507-31; 1999
2. Kubicka RA et al: A primer on the pulmonary vasculature. Med Radiogr Photogr 61:14-28, 1985
3. Fleischner FG et al: The butterfly pattern of acute pulmonary edema. Am J Cardiol 20:39-46, 1967

Eosinophilic Lung Disease

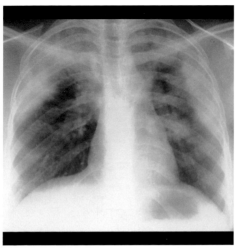

Chronic eosinophilic pneumonia. Bilateral peripheral consolidation in both upper lobes. Reverse "Bat's wing".

Key Facts
- Upper lobe peripheral homogeneous consolidation
- During resolution, nonanatomic wavy lines paralleling chest wall
- Fever, weight loss, nonanatomic cough
- Rapid resolution with steroids

Imaging Findings
<u>General Features</u>
- Best imaging clue: Chronic peripheral upper lobe consolidation

<u>Chest Radiograph</u>
- Chronic eosinophilic lung disease
  - Homogeneous peripheral consolidation predominately upper lung zones
    - "Reverse butterfly or photographic negative pulmonary edema"
  - Normal heart size: No pleural effusions or adenopathy
  - May wax and wane like simple eosinophilic pneumonia (Löffler's)
  - Resolution
    - Inner edge of peripheral consolidation may leave lines paralleling the chest wall
    - Rapid resolution with steroids
  - Recurrence: Same place, same size, same shape
- Simple eosinophilic pneumonia (Löffler's syndrome)
  - Migratory nonsegmental pulmonary consolidation
  - No pleural effusions or adenopathy
- Acute eosinophilic pneumonia
  - Diffuse mixed interstitial and alveolar opacities
  - Focal consolidation less common, no peripheral predominance
  - Small to moderate pleural effusions
  - No adenopathy
  - Marked resolution with steroid therapy
- Churg-Strauss syndrome
  - Migratory nonsegmental pulmonary consolidation

Eosinophilic Lung Disease

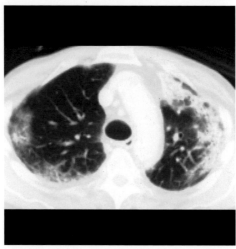

CT through upper lobes. Subpleural consolidation with sparing of the central portion of the lung. Chronic eosinophilic pneumonia. Differential includes BOOP and periarteritis nodosa.

- o Pleural effusions (1/3)
- o May have adenopathy
- Hypereosinophilic syndrome
  - o Patchy consolidation may be nodular or interstitial thickening
  - o May have pleural effusions
  - o Parenchymal changes from pulmonary embolus

CT/HRCT Findings
- More sensitive than chest radiograph, findings similar to radiograph
  - o May have mild mediastinal adenopathy or small pleural effusions

Imaging Recommendations
- Chest radiography usually sufficient for detection and follow-up

Differential Diagnosis

Bronchiolitis Obliterans Organizing Pneumonia (BOOP)
- May have identical radiographic findings, more likely lower lung zones

Aspiration
- Usually not as peripheral as chronic eosinophilic pneumonia

Pulmonary Embolus
- Usually associated with pleural effusions
- Infarcts are not as confluent as eosinophilic consolidation

Pathology

General
- Eosinophils derived from bone marrow, transient, half-life: 18 hrs
- Tissue eosinophilia may not have blood eosinophilia and vice versa
- Normal eosinophils in bronchoalveolar lavage < 1%, increased in eosinophilic lung disease

Microscopic Features
- Alveoli flooded with eosinophils, macrophages, and mononuclear cells

Eosinophilic Lung Disease

- Bronchiolitis obliterans in one-third; granulomas absent
- Churg-Strauss syndrome: Small vessel giant cell vasculitis

Clinical Issues
Presentation
- Eosinophilic lung disease
  - Diagnosis by
    - Peripheral eosinophilia with chest abnormalities
    - Tissue proven eosinophilic involvement
    - Eosinophils increased in bronchoalveolar lavage
  - Eosinophils increased in pleural fluid following pneumothorax, is not considered an eosinophilic lung disease
  - **Parasites** and **drugs** also cause eosinophilic lung disease
    - Drug induced: Sulfasalazine, penicillin, iodinated contrast, Dilantin, methotrexate, ibuprofen, tetracycline
- Chronic eosinophilic pneumonia
  - Cause unknown: Typically middle-aged women 2:1
  - 50% have history of asthma
  - Cough, significant weight loss, high fever, malaise, SOB, occasional hemoptysis, eosinophilia in 90% (conversely may be normal), pulmonary function test with mild restriction unless have asthma
- Simple eosinophilic pneumonia
  - Spontaneously resolves within 1 month, no treatment required
- Acute eosinophilic pneumonia
  - Acute respiratory failure requiring mechanical ventilation
  - Rapid onset, may have fever and myalgias
- Churg-Strauss syndrome
  - Asthma (history > 5 years); as asthma improves vasculitis worsens
  - Allergic rhinitis and paranasal sinus disease
  - Eosinophilia
  - Skin: Nodules, purpura
  - Systemic disease, other common involvement
    - GI: Abdominal pain 60%; diarrhea 33%; GI bleeding 20%
    - Cardiac: Heart failure (50%); pericarditis (33%)
    - Renal insufficiency (50%): Arthralgias (50%)
- Hypereosinophilic syndrome
  - Eosinophilia > 6 months (> 50% total white cell count)
  - Multiorgan involvement: Cardiac, peripheral neuropathy, GI tract, joints, skin, kidneys
  - Symptoms: Night sweats, anorexia, weight loss, pruritus, cough, fever
  - 2/3 develop thromboembolism
Treatment
- May spontaneously resolve without treatment
- Steroids, relapse common (50%) with discontinuation of steroids

Selected References
1. Allen JN et al: Eosinophilic lung diseases. Am J Respir Crit Care Med 150:1423-38, 1994
2. Mayo JR et al: Chronic eosinophilic pneumonia: CT findings in six cases. AJR 153:727-30, 1989
3. Gaensler EA et al: Peripheral opacities in chronic eosinophilic pneumonia: The photographic negative of pulmonary edema. AJR 128:1-13, 1977

Diffuse Alveolar Hemorrhage

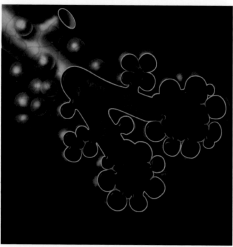

Alveolar hemorrhage. Hemosiderin laden macrophages within alveoli and interstitium promote clearing of blood. Repeated bouts of pulmonary hemorrhage will result in alveolar septal fibrosis.

Key Facts
- Edema pattern, acutely develop central-basilar consolidation
- Evolves to interstitial thickening over 3 days and clears over 12 days
- Etiology: Both immune and nonimmune
- Common causes: Goodpasture's, idiopathic pulmonary hemosiderosis, vasculitis, bone marrow transplantation (BMT)
- Iron deficiency anemia
- Hemoptysis in 80% (importantly may be absent)

Imaging Findings
General Features
- Best imaging clue: Basilar interstitial thickening or consolidation in anemic patient
Chest Radiograph
- Acutely develop basilar consolidation, resembles pulmonary edema
- Evolution
  - Consolidation evolves over 3 days into reticular interstitial thickening (including Kerley B lines)
  - Interstitial thickening resolves over 12 days
  - Repeated hemorrhage eventually interstitial thickening permanent
- May have small effusions
- Adenopathy may be seen in idiopathic pulmonary hemosiderosis (IPH)
CT/HRCT Findings
- More sensitive, acute hemorrhage opacities spectrum from focal ground glass to diffuse consolidation
- Subacute: 1-3 mm micronodules and interlobular septal thickening
MRI Findings
- Hemorrhage - intermediate signal T1
- Low signal T2 (iron susceptibility effect)

Diffuse Alveolar Hemorrhage

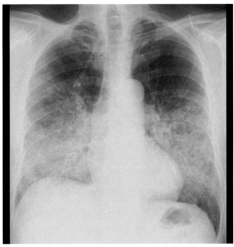

Diffuse alveolar hemorrhage in a patient with microscopic polyangitis. "Bat's wing" pattern of pulmonary consolidation is nonspecific. Normal heart size with cardiac pulmonary edema. Anemia often present but not hemoptysis.

<u>Imaging Recommendations</u>
- Chest radiographs usually sufficient to document extent of pathology and evolution over time

Differential Diagnosis
<u>Edema</u>
- Cardiomegaly
- Effusions more common
- Hemorrhage will not shift with gravity (gravitational shift test)

<u>Infection</u>
- Fever
- Will not have evolution from consolidation to interstitial pattern
- Consolidation or interstitial pattern may be similar

Pathology
<u>General</u>
- General path comments
  - Flooding alveolar spaces with blood
  - Hemosiderin-laden macrophages, key finding in bronchoalveolar lavage
  - Chronic: Additional septal fibrosis
- Etiology
  - Immune mediated
    - Anti-glomerular basement membrane disease (AGBMD): Goodpasture's
    - Glomerulonephritis
    - Systemic lupus erythematosus
    - Wegener's
    - Vasculitis
    - Henoch-Schönlein purpura

Diffuse Alveolar Hemorrhage

- Idiopathic pulmonary hemosiderosis (IPH)
  - o Nonimmune
    - Bleeding diathesis: Disseminated intravascular coagulation (DIC); anticoagulation (rare)
    - Leukemia
    - Bone marrow transplantation (implantation response)
    - Mitral stenosis
    - Uremia, severe
- Pathophysiology
  - o Hemorrhage into airspaces (consolidation)
  - o Blood removed from alveoli by macrophages (3 days)
  - o Macrophages migrate into interstitium (interstitial thickening)
  - o Macrophages removed by lymphatics (clearing 12 days)

Clinical Issues
Presentation
- Nonspecific cough, dyspnea
- Hemoptysis not as frequent as anticipated (80%)
- Iron deficiency anemia
- IPH
  - o Children or young men
- AGBMD
  - o May follow influenza-like illness
  - o Young men
- Systemic lupus erythematosus (SLE)
  - o Facial rash
  - o Young women
- BMT
  - o Temporally correlated with engraftment of bone marrow

Treatment
- Immune complex disease
  - o Immunosuppression
  - o Steroids
  - o Plasmapheresis

Prognosis
- Depends on etiology

Selected References
1. Witte RJ et al: Diffuse pulmonary alveolar hemorrhage after bone marrow transplantation: Radiographic findings in 39 patients. AJR 157:461-4, 1991
2. Albelda SM et al: Diffuse pulmonary hemorrhage: A review and classification. Radiology 154:289-97, 1985
3. Bowley NB et al: The chest X-ray in antiglomerular basement membrane antibody disease (Goodpasture's syndrome). Clin Radiol 30:419-29, 1979

Neurogenic Pulmonary Edema

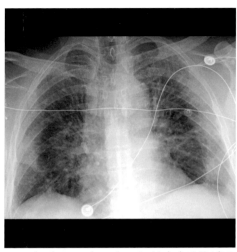

Acute CVA neurogenic pulmonary edema. In contrast to hydrostatic edema, neurogenic edema atypical. Asymmetric peripheral pulmonary edema and small pleural effusions.

Key Facts
- Any CNS injury (including seizures) that increases intracranial pressure (ICP)
- Capillary stress failure, edema based on both hydrostatic mechanisms and capillary leak
- Radiographically, edema pattern asymmetric, often upper lung zone predominant

Imaging Findings
General Features
- Best imaging clue: Atypical pulmonary edema patterns after CNS insult

Chest Radiograph
- Onset acute (minutes) or subacute (12 hours) following CNS insult
- Edema pattern often asymmetric, often upper lobe or right side predominant
- Resolves over 24-48 hours

Other Imaging Modality
- Cranial CT or MRI useful to evaluate etiology

Imaging Recommendations
- Chest radiography: Clue to diagnosis; implies increased intracranial pressure, review neuroimaging studies; often a diagnosis of exclusion once contusion, aspiration, pneumonia excluded

Differential Diagnosis
Aspiration
- May be predominately upper lobes in supine comatose patient (gravitational segments posterior segments upper lobes)
- Aspiration extremely common with CNS insults, resolves more slowly than neurogenic pulmonary edema (NPE)

Neurogenic Pulmonary Edema

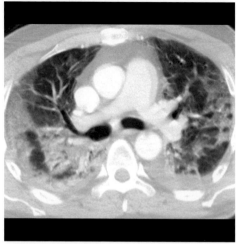

Neurogenic pulmonary edema often has atypical features such as predominant peripheral or upper lobe distribution. Heart is usually normal in size.

Cardiogenic Pulmonary Edema
- Usually not predominately upper lobe
- Cardiomegaly
- Pleural effusions

Pneumonia
- Identical radiographic findings
- Often associated with fever

Contusion
- Immediately following trauma
- Motor vehicle accidents could give rise to both contusions and NPE

High Altitude Pulmonary Edema
- Similar radiographic pattern
- Seen with ascent > 5000 feet
- CNS insults from Acute Mountain Sickness may result in High Altitude Pulmonary Edema

Smoke Inhalation
- Similar radiographic pattern
- May have carbonaceous particles in sputum
- Develops within few hours of smoke inhalation

Mitral Regurgitant Pulmonary Edema
- Mitral regurgitant pulmonary edema predominant in right upper lobe
- Cardiomegaly

Pathology

General
- Pulmonary edema with features of both hydrostatic edema and capillary leak edema
- Etiology-pathogenesis-pathophysiology
  - Known features important in pathogenesis
    - Increased intracranial pressure effects mediated by spinal cord (NPE blocked with cord transection)

Neurogenic Pulmonary Edema

- "Sympathetic storm" (NPE blocked by alpha-adrenergic blocking agents – phentolamine)
- o Pulmonary venoconstriction and vascular mediators (not clearly defined) lead to capillary stress failure
- o Edema has features of both hydrostatic (pulmonary venoconstriction) and capillary leak

Clinical Issues

Presentation

- May result from any CNS injury that leads to increased ICP, includes seizure activity
- 50% incidence in head trauma
- Nonspecific signs: Tachycardia, tachypnea
- Fever common
- Hypoxia
- Protein rich sputum (due to capillary leak)

Treatment

- Supportive
- Oxygen, mechanical ventilation: Positive end-expiratory pressure (PEEP)
- Alpha-adrenergic blocking agents early, benefit unproven
- Dilantin or other anticonvulsants for seizures

Prognosis

- Depends on successful treatment of CNS cause

Selected References
1. Ell SR: Neurogenic pulmonary edema. A review of the literature and a perspective. Invest Radiol 26:499-506, 1991
2. West JB et al: Stress failure in pulmonary capillaries. J Appl Physiol 70:1731-42, 1991
3. Felman AH: Neurogenic pulmonary edema. Observations in 6 patients. AJR 112: 393-6, 1971

Lipoid Pneumonia

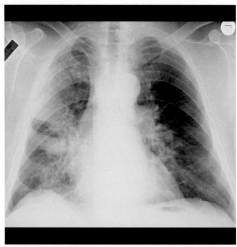

Chronic consolidation in the right mid and lower lung slowly progressed over 7 years. Differential for chronic consolidation includes lipoid pneumonia, BOOP, eosinophilic pneumonia, bronchioloalveolar cell carcinoma and lymphoma.

Key Facts
- Aspiration of oily substances, such as mineral oil, oil-based nose drops or Vicks VapoRub
- History of lipid use may be difficult to elicit from patient
- Radiographically, may be incidental finding of single or multiple irregular areas of consolidation in dependent lung
- Diagnosis can be made with CT by demonstrating fatty tissue attenuation
- Lipid-laden macrophages may be seen in bronchioalveolar lavage (BAL) fluid
- Patient usually asymptomatic but may have chronic cough
- Transthoracic needle biopsy can provide definitive diagnosis

Imaging Findings
General Features
- Best imaging clue: Low attenuation areas (~-100 HU) in consolidation at CT
- Early
    - Airspace opacification, confluent or discrete with air bronchograms
    - May be large areas with stellate or well-defined margins
    - In dependent lung, often segmental and in lower lobes
    - In debilitated patients – in posterior segments of upper lobes and superior segments of lower lobes
- Chronic
    - Multifocal basal mass-like areas of consolidation with irregular margins
    - Cicatricial volume loss in affected areas
    - Interstitial pattern to consolidation
    - Well-circumscribed peripheral mass
    - Gravity-dependent lung segments

Lipoid Pneumonia

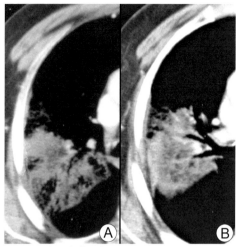

Sequential CT images (A and B) in the same patient. Several foci of consolidated lung were of low density (-95 HU). On questioning the patient had used oily nose drops for many years. Diagnosis: lipoid pneumonia. Note that in this patient with chronic aspiration, the majority of the aspirate went to the right lung.

CT Findings
- Diagnosis made with CT when the opacities show fatty attenuation (−50 to −150 HU)
- Lesions may have foci of ossification
- Lipoid etiology not apparent when interstitial pattern predominates
- Mixed ground-glass and interlobular septal thickening may simulate alveolar proteinosis
- Fat may shift to dependent lung with postural change

MR Findings
- MR may show fat: High T1 and T2 signal or chemical shift

Imaging Recommendations
- CT to investigate chronic alveolar disease
  o Fat density in lipoid pneumonia

Differential Diagnosis

Hamartoma
- May have fatty attenuation with CT; usually solitary mass, < 4 cm and may have popcorn calcification

Inflammatory Pseudotumor
- No fat attenuation, otherwise may have identical radiographic findings

Bronchiolitis Obliterans-Organizing Pneumonia (BOOP)
- Multifocal peripheral pulmonary consolidation, no fat attenuation

Bronchogenic Carcinoma
- Identical radiographic findings for solitary mass
- Cavitated carcinoma may have low attenuation material but not of fat density

Alveolar Proteinosis
- No fat attenuation; "crazy paving" pattern of alveolar proteinosis can be seen with lipoid pneumonia

Lipoid Pneumonia

Pathology
General
- Mixed inflammatory cells containing numerous lipid-laden macrophages
- Etiology-pathogenesis-pathophysiology
  - Mineral oil is most common agent, but may occur with animal or vegetable oils
  - Initial reaction is a bronchopneumonia; macrophages ingest the lipid
  - Clearing occurs by mucociliary transport or macrophage migration via the interstitium and lymphatics to mediastinal lymph nodes
  - Giant cell or granuloma formation may occur
  - With mineral oil aspiration, there are oil droplets within multinucleated giant cells, lymphocytes and fibrous tissue

Gross Pathologic-Surgical Features
- Chronically, lipid is fibrogenic, affected lung distorted and shrunken

Microscopic
- Hallmark is lipid-laden macrophages

Clinical Issues
Presentation
- Aspiration of oil used as a lubricant in infants with feeding problems
- Aspiration of mineral oil used for constipation in elderly
- Neurological or esophageal disease may promote aspiration
- Oil not irritant, aspiration often "silent"
- Most patients are asymptomatic and do not offer history of lipid use
- Commonly discovered as an incidental radiographic abnormality
- May have acute pneumonia with large amount of aspirated material
- Chronic cough
- Diagnosis by recovering lipid-laden macrophages in BAL fluid or transthoracic needle biopsy
- Radiographic findings may disappear with discontinuation of use of lipoid agent

Treatment
- Small amount aspirated – little impairment
- Large amounts – may develop restrictive lung disease or cor pulmonale
- May increase risk for bronchogenic carcinoma and nontuberculous mycobacterial infection

Selected References
1. Seo JB et al: Shark liver oil-induced lipoid pneumonia in pigs: Correlation of thin-section CT and histopathologic findings. Radiology 212:88-96, 1999
2. Van den Plas O et al: Gravity-dependent infiltrates in a patient with lipoid pneumonia. Chest 98:1253-4, 1990
3. Wheeler et al: Diagnosis of lipoid pneumonia by computed tomography. JAMA 245:65-6, 1981

Viral Pneumonia

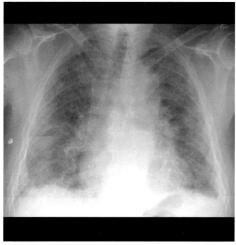

Viral pneumonia. Nonspecific diffuse interstitial and ground glass opacities. Borderline cardiomegaly.

Key Facts
- Respiratory syncytial virus most common viral pneumonia in children
- Influenza most common viral pneumonia in adults
- Variable radiographic pattern, commonly diffuse and nodular
- Usually involves small airways leading to
  - Bronchial wall thickening
  - Air trapping or
  - Subsegmental atelectasis
- Rare late complication: Bronchiolitis obliterans

Imaging Findings
<u>General Features</u>
- Best imaging clue: Diffuse interstitial thickening in febrile patient
<u>Chest Radiograph</u>
- Diffuse interstitial thickening or patchy consolidation
  - Small pleural effusions, uncommon
  - Small airways disease
    - Bronchial wall thickening
    - Air trapping common or
    - Subsegmental atelectasis
  - No cavities
  - Hemorrhagic pulmonary edema: Hantavirus
- Focal disease uncommon
- Hilar adenopathy
  - Rare, limits differential: Measles; infectious mononucleosis
  - Complications
    - Predisposed to bacterial superinfection
    - Bronchiolitis obliterans late finding
<u>CT Findings</u>
- More sensitive than chest radiography

Viral Pneumonia

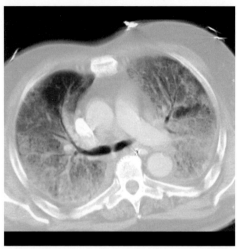

Viral pneuomonia. Diffuse ground glass opacities nonspecific. Differential includes edema or hemorrhage.

Imaging Recommendations
- Chest radiography: Usually sufficient for documenting pattern and extent of disease and to monitor therapy
- CT: More sensitive, may be important in immunocompromised patients to document disease and begin early treatment

Differential Diagnosis
Edema
- Edema will evolve quickly and resolve with diuretics
- Interstitial thickening will change with position (gravitational shift test)
Hemorrhage
- Anemia with hemorrhage, often hemoptysis
- Identical radiographic findings
- Often evolves from consolidation to interstitial thickening
Aspiration
- Identical radiographic findings
- Often recurrent, viral pneumonias tend not to be recurrent
Bronchiolitis Obliterans-Organizing Pneumonia (BOOP)
- Multifocal areas of peripheral pulmonary consolidation
- Often waxes and wanes, unusual evolution with viral pneumonia
Farmer's Lung
- Farmer's lung often mistaken as pneumonia: Also tends to be recurrent with repeated exposure to offending antigen
Alveolar Proteinosis
- "Bat's wing" central consolidation
- Patients often asymptomatic in contrast to patients with viral pneumonia

Pathology
General
- Mixed inflammatory cells, predominately lymphocytic in airspaces or interstitium

Viral Pneumonia

- Etiology-pathogenesis-pathophysiology
  - Portal of entry: Inhalation
  - Most common viruses: Influenza, respiratory syncytial virus (RSV), infectious mononucleosis (Epstein-Barr virus), herpes simplex, varicella-zoster, adenovirus, measles, cytomegalovirus (CMV), Hantavirus
  - Offending organism rarely cultured
  - Bronchiolitis in small airways
    - Sloughing ciliated cells
    - Bronchial wall thickening and edema
    - Lymphocytic infiltration interstitium: Multinucleated giant cells highly specific for measles
    - Bronchiolitis obliterans late

Clinical Issues

Presentation

- Nonspecific symptoms: Fever, dry cough, myalgias, headaches, rhinitis, pharyngitis
- Respiratory physical exam may be normal
- Common cause of confusion in adults
- Specific virus
  - Influenza A, B, C
    - Epidemics, most common viral pneumonia adults
    - Late winter most common
  - RSV
    - Most common viral pneumonia in infants and children
    - Winter most common
  - Infectious mononucleosis: Pneumonia rare; large spleen
  - Herpes simplex: AIDS highly susceptible; associated with oral ulcers
  - Varicella-zoster
    - Pneumonia uncommon in children
    - Heals with miliary calcifications similar to histoplasmosis
  - Adenovirus: Common; most common etiology of bronchiolitis obliterans
  - Measles: Uncommon; may have adenopathy
  - CMV: Immunocompromised, cell mediated defect; reactivation of latent infection
  - Hantavirus
    - Southwest, arid, aerosols of urine infected deer mouse
    - Rapidly fatal

Treatment

- Preventive: Influenza vaccine, measles vaccine, varicella vaccine
- Supportive
- Acyclovir for varicella or herpes: Ganciclovir for CMV

Prognosis

- Variable depending on virulence of virus and host response

Selected References
1. Scanlon GT et al: The radiology of bacterial and viral pneumonias. Radiol Clin North Am 11:317-38, 1973
2. Conte P et al: Viral pneumonia. Roentgen pathological correlations. Radiology 95:267-72, 1970

Pneumonia

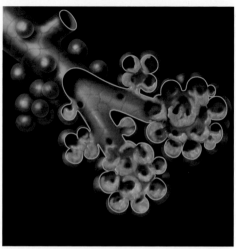

Bacterial pneumonia. Inflammatory exudate begins in distal air spaces and spreads to adjacent segments through the pores of Kohn. Air-filled airways surrounded by consolidated lung are visualized as air bronchograms.

Key Facts
- Diagnosis based on culture
- Absence of parenchymal abnormality excludes pneumonia (except in immunocompromised)
- Pattern not diagnostic of organism, single organism may cause multiple patterns

Imaging Findings
General Features
- Best imaging clue: Focal parenchymal abnormality in patient with fever

Chest Radiograph
- High sensitivity
  - Exceptions, may not have visible abnormality in
    - Immunocompromised patients, especially if neutropenic
    - Dehydration: Controversial; rare if it exists at all
- Nearly any pattern from consolidation to interstitial thickening
- Lobar vs. bronchopneumonia
  - Pathologic designation rarely helpful radiographically
  - Difficult to reliably identify (poor interobserver agreement)
- Hilar adenopathy
  - Rare, limits differential: Tuberculosis, mycoplasma, fungi, mononucleosis, measles, plague, tularemia, anthrax, pertussis
- Parapneumonic effusion vs. empyema
  - Loculation suggests empyema
  - Simple effusions in patients with previous adhesions also loculated
- Pneumatoceles
  - Develop later in course of pneumonia (classically Staph aureus)
  - Develop later and persist for months, usually spontaneously resolve
- Complications: Empyema, abscess, bronchopleural fistula
- Resolution

Pneumonia

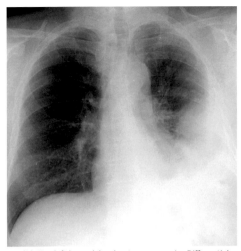

Extensive consolidation left lower lobe due to pneumonia. Differential would include infarct or hemorrhage.

- o Delayed with advancing age and involvement of multiple lobes
  - ▪ Faster resolution in nonsmokers and outpatients
- o Time table, expected
  - ▪ 50% resolution 2 weeks; 66% 4 weeks; 75% 6 weeks

CT Findings
- Utility to detect complications, especially empyemas
- Separate abscess from empyema
  - o Abscess: Thick, irregular wall; round, small contact with chest wall
  - o Empyema: Thin, uniform wall; lenticular, broad contact with chest, split pleura sign
- Evaluate cause in patients with recurrent pneumonia
  - o Recurrent pneumonias consider
    - ▪ Bronchogenic carcinoma, bronchiectasis, tracheobronchomegaly, COPD, pulmonary alveolar proteinosis, sequestration, esophageal diverticulum, right middle lobe syndrome

Imaging Recommendations
- Chest radiograph: Usually sufficient for detection and monitor therapy
- CT
  - o Useful in immunocompromised with normal chest radiographs
  - o More sensitive and specific for complications
  - o Useful to screen for underlying structural abnormalities such as bronchiectasis or occult endobronchial obstruction

Differential Diagnosis
Edema
- Cardiomegaly and pulmonary venous hypertension
- Edema will shift with position (gravitational shift test)
Hemorrhage
- Patients usually anemic and often have hemoptysis

Pneumonia

Aspiration
• May have predisposing condition such as esophageal motility disorder
Bronchiolitis Obliterans-Organizing Pneumonia (BOOP)
• Patients often treated for pneumonia for variable length of time
Chronic Eosinophilic Pneumonia
• Typically peripheral upper lobe consolidation
• Will not respond to antibiotics
Farmer's Lung
• Farmer's lung often mistaken as pneumonia
• History of antigen exposure
Infarcts
• Resolution – infarcts "melting snowball" sign, pneumonia fades
Atelectasis
• Fissural displacement or other signs of air loss

Pathology
General
• Offending organism cultured in < 50%
• Portal of entry inhalation or aspiration oral secretions
Gross Pathologic-Surgical Features
• Lobar vs. bronchopneumonia
  o Lobar
    ▪ Alveolar flooding with inflammatory exudate, especially neutrophils
    ▪ Rapidly spreads throughout lobe, only stopped by intact fissures
    ▪ Usually peripheral in lung
  o Bronchopneumonia
    ▪ Exudate centered on terminal bronchioles (centriacinar)
    ▪ Respects septal boundaries
    ▪ Patchy – adjacent lobules may be normal, patchwork quilt pattern
Microscopic Features
• Nonspecific acute and/or chronic inflammatory cells
• Organism identification with special stains (Gram or acid-fast)

Clinical Issues
Presentation
• 5th leading cause of death
• Fever, chills, cough, sputum production
• Empyema - may be surprisingly free of toxic symptoms
• Pulmonary cavity in edentulous patients = lung cancer
• Consolidation + bacteremia = pneumonia
Treatment
• Appropriate antibiotics
• Drain empyemas, not abscesses
• Bronchoscopy for recurrent disease in same location
Prognosis
• Depends on virulence of organism, antibiotic susceptibility and host

Selected References
1. Geppert EF: Recurrent pneumonia. Chest 98: 739-45, 1990
2. Scanlon GT et al: The radiology of bacterial and viral pneumonias. Radiol Clin North Am 11:317-38, 1973

Fungal Pneumonia

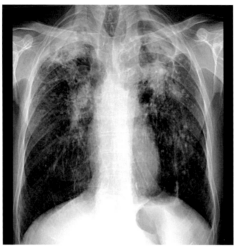

Extensive biapical fibrosis, pleural thickening, and volume loss from previous silicosis. Large mycetoma left apex, suspect mycetoma right apex.

Key Facts
- Common, self-limited, asymptomatic infection
- Most related to spores inhaled from nitrogen-rich (from bird excreta) soil
- Acute pneumonia: Focal pneumonia with enlarged lymph nodes
- Chronic progressive: Upper lobe cavitary disease mimics tuberculosis
- Dissemination: Miliary lung and other organ involvement

Imaging Findings
General Features
- Best imaging clue: High index of suspicion in patients from endemic areas
Chest Radiograph
- Acute primary pneumonia
  - Variable-sized, single foci of consolidation or multiple nodules
  - Regional hilar and mediastinal adenopathy common
- Chronic progressive pneumonia: Mimics post primary tuberculosis
- Disseminated: Widespread consolidation or miliary nodules
- Healed primary pneumonia: Granuloma (Ghon lesion)
  - Time to calcify variable: 6 months (children) to years (adults)
  - Patterns: Central nidus, laminated, diffuse, miliary
  - Satellite nodules common
- Histoplasmosis
  - Acute primary pneumonia: Residual punctate calcification in liver and spleen
- Blastomycosis
  - Acute primary pneumonia: Large central pulmonary mass mimics bronchogenic carcinoma → scattered nodules: Mimic metastases
- Coccidioidomycosis
  - Acute primary pneumonia: Residual thin-walled cavities (5%) → upper lung zone predominate; pleural effusions (5%)
- Cryptococcosis (torulosis): Small subpleural nodule(s)
- Aspergillosis

Fungal Pneumonia

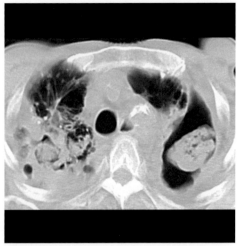

Large mycetoma left upper lobe cavity. Smaller mycetomas right apex. Mycetomas may contain air and even calcium.

- o Allergic bronchopulmonary aspergillosis: Fleeting subsegmental consolidation; central bronchiectasis, mucoid impactions primarily upper lobes
- o Aspergilloma (fungus ball): Positionally dependent intracavitary mass; CT: Sponge-like filling of cavity precedes mycetoma
- o Chronic necrotizing or semi-invasive: Mimics post primary tuberculosis
- o Invasive aspergillosis: CT halo sign → large, dense, central nidus, thin rim, ground-glass opacity, (early); air crescent sign (late); coincidental with rising neutrophil count and good prognosis
- Candidiasis
  - o Diffuse pneumonia: Often superimposed on edema or infection
- Sporotrichosis: Chronic progressive disease only

Imaging Recommendations
- Radiographs usually sufficient for detection and therapy: CT often helpful in halo sign and aspergillomas

Differential Diagnosis
Acute Primary Pneumonia or Disseminated
- Other pneumonia: Requires culture
- Hemorrhage: Identical radiographic findings, patients anemic
- Aspiration: Identical radiographic findings
- Contusion: Follows blunt chest trauma, resolves over 10-14 days
- Pulmonary edema: Cardiomegaly and pleural effusion
- Farmer's lung: History of exposure to inhaled antigen
- Bronchioloalveolar cell carcinoma: Progressive, doesn't resolve
- Alveolar proteinosis: Central "bat's-wing"

Miliary Calcification
- Healed chickenpox pneumonia

Chronic Progressive Pneumonia
- Post primary tuberculosis: Requires culture
- Chronic eosinophilic pneumonia: Peripheral consolidation

- Ankylosing spondylitis: Spinal changes of ankylosing spondylitis

Pathology
<u>General</u>
- 2-6 week incubation period
- Histoplasmosis: Yeast clustered within histiocyte
- Blastomycosis: Large, broad-necked bud
- Coccidioidomycosis: Giant spherule packed with endospores
- Cryptococcosis: Large capsule
- Aspergillosis: Septated hyphae with 45^0 branching
- Candida: Yeast with pseudohyphae
- Sporotrichosis: Mickey mouse ear buds

Clinical Issues
<u>Presentation</u>
- Most infections asymptomatic: Nonspecific malaise, cough, weight loss
- Specific fungi
  - Histoplasmosis
    - Geography: River valleys (Mississippi); source: Bird excreta soil
    - Symptoms generally seen with massive point exposure; radiograph often worse than clinical impression
  - Blastomycosis
    - Geography: Southeastern US, Great Lakes; source: Unknown
    - Skin (66%): Face, upper extremities, mimics basal cell carcinoma
    - Bone (33%): Intervertebral disc infection, mimics tuberculosis
    - Genitourinary (20%): Prostate, epididymis
    - If untreated tends to recur within 3 years
  - Coccidioidomycosis
    - Geography: Desert semi-arid (Southwestern US); source: Soil
    - Erythema nodosum (20%), arthritis (20%)
  - Cryptococcosis
    - Geography: Worldwide; source: Pigeon excreta-enriched soil
    - Meningitis most common presentation
  - Aspergillosis
    - Geography: Worldwide; source: Soil
    - Allergic bronchopulmonary aspergillosis: Asthma, eosinophilia
    - Aspergilloma: Hemoptysis, symptoms from pre-existing cavity
  - Candidiasis
    - Geography: Worldwide; source: Normal GI flora
    - Immunosuppressed patients on broad spectrum antibiotics
  - Sporotrichosis
    - Geography: Worldwide; source: Roses, sphagnum moss
    - Localized skin lesion with regional adenopathy
<u>Treatment</u>
- Often self-limited: Amphotericin B or Ketoconazole for severe infection (K iodide for sporotrichosis)

Selected References
1. Mcadams HP et al: Thoracic mycoses from endemic fungi: Radiologic-pathologic correlation. Radiographics 15: 255-70, 1995
2. Mcadams HP et al: Thoracic mycoses from opportunistic fungi: Radiologic-pathologic correlation. Radiographics 15: 271-86, 1995

Pulmonary Alveolar Proteinosis

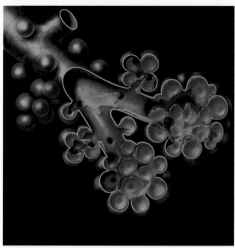

Pulmonary alveolar proteinosis. Alveolar filling with lipid-rich proteinaceous material that resembles surfactant. May be due to proliferation and desquamation of type II pneumocytes and/or reduced clearance by defective macrophages.

Key Facts
- Accumulation of abundant protein-rich and lipid-rich surfactant material in alveoli
- Radiographically, bilateral symmetric central airspace opacities or vague, hazy opacities, perihilar and in lower lungs
- HRCT shows a "crazy-paving" appearance
- A third of patients are asymptomatic
- Occurs with massive silica dust exposure
- Associated with infections such as Nocardia
- Diagnosed and treated with bronchioloalveolar lavage (BAL) and irrigation
- Good prognosis

Imaging Findings
General Features
- Best imaging clue: "Crazy paving" pattern at HRCT

Chest Radiograph
- Chronic consolidation, may be nodular
- Central perihilar "bat's wing" pattern
- Mixed interstitial and airspace opacities, less common

CT Findings
- HRCT shows geographic regions of airspace or ground glass opacities and linear interstitial opacities, giving a "crazy-paving" pattern
- Distribution of disease is random

Imaging Recommendations
- Chest radiography: Usually sufficient to document extent of disease and monitor therapy
- CT
  - Useful for diagnosis
  - More sensitive to screen for complications such as opportunistic infection

Pulmonary Alveolar Proteinosis

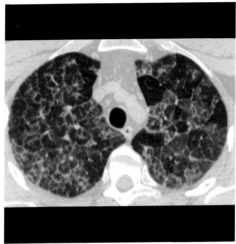

HRCT pulmonary alveolar proteinosis. Crazy paving pattern. Septal thickening and ground glass opacities in a geographic distribution.

Differential Diagnosis

Pulmonary Edema
- "Bat's-wing" pattern in patient with cardiomegaly and pulmonary venous hypertension
- Pleural effusions uncommon with pulmonary alveolar proteinosis (PAP)

Pneumonia
- Usually not asymptomatic
- Positive cultures

Hemorrhage
- Patients usually have anemia and may have hemoptysis
- Radiographic findings may be identical

Bronchioloalveolar Cell Carcinoma
- May have identical radiographic pattern

"Crazy-Paving" Pattern
- Also seen in bronchioloalveolar carcinoma, lipoid pneumonia, hemorrhage, pulmonary edema and bacterial pneumonia

Pathology

General
- Accumulation of abundant protein rich and lipid rich surfactant material
- Etiology-pathogenesis-pathophysiology
    - Abnormality of surfactant production, metabolism, or clearance by type II alveolar cells and macrophages
    - Often superinfected with Nocardia, Aspergillus, Cryptococcus and other organisms
    - May occur with exposure to high concentrations of silicon dioxide dust or titanium
    - May occur in immunocompromised children, or adults with lymphoma, leukemia, AIDS, or autoimmune disease

Pulmonary Alveolar Proteinosis

Microscopic Features
- Alveoli are filled with fine granular material that stains pink with PAS stain

Clinical Issues
Presentation
- Uncommon
- Adults 20 to 50 years olds, may occur in young children
- >2:1 male predominance
- Chest radiograph is abnormal out of proportion to patient's symptoms
- 33% are asymptomatic, most common symptoms are dyspnea and cough
- Clubbing of fingers and toes
- Diagnosis with BAL or transbronchial biopsy

Treatment
- Therapeutic BAL with whole lung irrigation, usually one to two times; few patients require annual or biannual therapeutic BALs

Prognosis
- Good
- Death from pulmonary fibrosis is rare

Selected References
1. Murch CR et al: Computed tomography appearances of pulmonary alveolar proteinosis. Clin Radiol 40:240-43, 1989
2. Prakash UB et al: Pulmonary alveolar phospholipoproteinosis: Experience with 34 cases and a review. Mayo Clin 62: 499-518, 1987
3. Gale ME et al: Bronchopulmonary lavage in pulmonary alveolar proteinosis: Chest radiograph observations. AJR 146:981-5, 1986

Toxic Inhalation

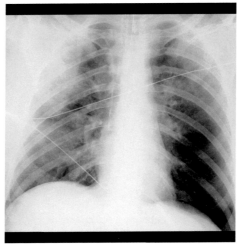

Smoke Inhalation. Diffuse consolidation predominantly peripheral and upper lobes. Intubated. Pattern of smoke inhalation often atypical and more severely affects the upper lobes.

Key Facts
- Noncardiac edema due to chemical injury from toxic inhalation
- Early radiographic findings: Perihilar bronchial wall thickening and subglottic edema
- Late: Hemorrhagic pulmonary edema (smoke: Predominately upper lobes)
- Superimposed pneumonia common complication
- Late onset bronchiolitis obliterans (rare)

Imaging Findings
General Features
- Best imaging clue: Diffuse pulmonary edema following toxic fume inhalation
Chest Radiograph
- Earliest radiographic manifestation: Bronchial wall thickening and subglottic edema
- Onset: Immediate to first 24 hours
- Severity dependent on concentration and length of exposure
- Location: Predominately perihilar and upper lung zone in smoke inhalation
- Resolves over 3-5 days
- Pleural effusions may develop without parenchymal abnormality, probably related to hypoproteinemia from skin burns
- Normal heart size
- Bronchiolitis obliterans, rare, weeks to months later
  - Ill-defined, small nodules in previously affected lung
  - Hyperinflation
Xenon-133 Ventilation Scanning
- Air trapping and delayed washout
- Maybe abnormal when chest radiograph normal
- Rarely used

Toxic Inhalation

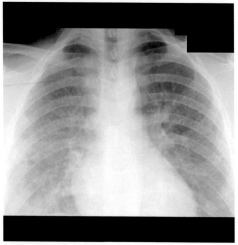

Silo-fillers disease. Working in freshly filled silo. Became dyspneic 4 hours later. Diffuse micronodular interstitial thickening.

<u>Imaging Recommendations</u>
- Chest radiographs suffice for extent of injury and monitoring course

Differential Diagnosis
<u>Fluid Overload</u>
- Identical radiographic findings
- Fluid overload common due to massive fluid administration for skin burns
<u>Pneumonia</u>
- Identical radiographic findings
- Superimposed pneumonia common, develops 48 hours after admission
- Any worsening of consolidation after 48 hours should be considered superinfection
<u>Atelectasis</u>
- Signs of volume loss
- Atelectasis common due to mucosal airway injury with edema and narrowing and ciliary injury with impaired clearance of secretions
<u>Aspiration</u>
- Identical radiographic findings and similar course
<u>In Agricultural Workers</u>
- Farmer's lung
  - Similar radiographic findings, may be nodular in contrast to toxic fume inhalation
  - Usually seen in the spring from moldy dust silage, silo-filler's disease in fall
- Organic dust toxicity syndrome: Radiographs usually normal

Pathology
<u>General</u>
- Severity of chemical pneumonitis dependent on composition and concentration of smoke and length of exposure

Toxic Inhalation

- o Injury may occur from upper airways to pulmonary capillary bed
- o Smoke inhalation
    - Numerous gaseous oxides produced when wood and plastic burn
    - Chemical pneumonitis from gases, thermal injury rare
- o Silo-filler's disease
    - Inhalation of nitrogen dioxide (NO_2)
    - Green forage crops undergo fermentation by aerobic bacteria: Oxidation leads to NO and the NO_2; orange-brown gas with strong odor similar to ammonia or chlorine; NO_2 combines with water in lung to produce nitrous acid, injuring epithelium
- Pathophysiology
    - o Toxic gas concentrations dependent on V/Q ratio
    - o Normal upright lung, V/Q ratio highest in upper lung zone

Gross Pathologic Features
- Acute injury results in hemorrhagic pulmonary edema, proteinaceous fluid exudates and hyaline membrane formation
- Chronically, small airways damage results in bronchiolitis obliterans

Microscopic Pathology
- Acutely, diffuse alveolar damage with hyaline membrane formation
- Chronically, bronchiolitis obliterans

Clinical Issues

Presentation
- Nonspecific respiratory distress following smoke inhalation
- Immediate symptoms, cough, light-headedness, dyspnea
- Delayed symptoms months later: Dyspnea, nonproductive cough
- Wheezing common due to airway injury
- Carbonaceous sputum in smoke inhalation
- Elevated carboxyhemoglobin (from carbon monoxide inhalation)
- Bronchoscopic findings in smoke inhalation
    - o Laryngeal edema
    - o Airway ulceration, necrosis, charring depending on severity

Treatment
- Supportive, mechanical ventilation: Positive End-Expiratory Pressure (PEEP)
- Serial cultures for infectious surveillance
- Steroids may be helpful
- Preventive: Avoid freshly-filled silo for 14 days (gases dissipate a few weeks after ensilage)
    - o NO_2 also formed during welding and operation Zamboni machines

Prognosis
- Variable, depends on extent of initial injury

Selected References
1. Gurney JW et al: Agricultural disorders of the lung. Radiographics 11: 625-34, 1991
2. Lee MJ et al: The plain chest radiograph after acute smoke inhalation. Clin Radiol 39:33-7, 1988
3. Teixidor HS et al: Smoke inhalation: Radiologic manifestations. Radiology 149:383-7, 1983

Immunocompromised Host

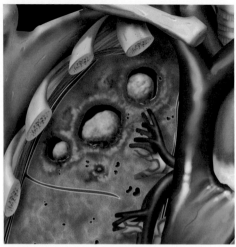

Invasive aspergillosis in neutropenic patient with leukemia. Crescentic cavities form as the neutrophil count improves. Peripheral "halo" sign represents hemorrhagic edema. Similar appearance is seen with invasive mucormycosis.

Key Facts
- Lung main focus of complications in immunocompromised host
- 75% of all complications are infections
- Up to 1/3rd have more than 1 complication
- Statistics don't substitute for sampling
- Types of complications
  - Infection, edema, hemorrhage, underlying disease, drug and radiation reaction, graft vs. host disease (GVHD)

Imaging Findings
General Features
- Radiologic diagnostic interpretations correct in 1/3rd
- Accuracy of highly confident diagnosis 50% (toss up)
- Sensitivity probably > 90%
- Utility
  - Surveillance prior to onset symptoms, detection, evolution, complications, monitor response to therapy

Chest Radiograph
- Consolidation
  - Focal or diffuse, subsegmental to diffuse, consider
    - Bacterial, mycobacteria, fungal: Hemorrhage, radiation therapy, lymphoma
- Nodules, consider
  - Fungal, nocardia, mycobacteria: Septic emboli, metastases, bleomycin toxicity, post-transplant lymphoproliferative disorder (PTLD)
- Interstitial, consider
  - PCP, virus: Edema, cardiac and noncardiac (Kerley B lines more likely due to edema than infection), drug reaction, lymphangitic tumor
- Pleural effusion, consider
  - CHF: Bacterial pneumonia, infarct, GVHD

48

Immunocompromised Host

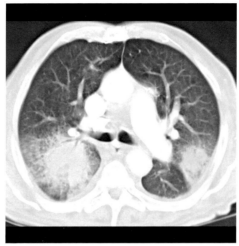

CT. Airspace masses have large dense nidus surrounded by halo of ground glass opacity. Diagnosis: Invasive aspergillosis in neutropenic patient diagnosed with leukemia.

CT Findings
- HRCT inspiration and expiration for bronchiolitis obliterans
  - Mosaic perfusion with air trapping at expiration
- Specific conditions such as invasive aspergillosis discussed elsewhere

Imaging Recommendations
- Chest radiography usually sufficient for clinical practice; CT more sensitive, will detect infection an average of 5 days before chest radiograph abnormalities

Differential Diagnosis
- None

Pathology
General
- Type of immunosuppression
  - Mechanical
    - Mucosal disruption (chemotherapy), intubation (bypass nose and airway defenses), splenectomy
  - Cellular
    - Macrophages, neutrophil dysfunction: B-cell or T-cell dysfunction
- Etiology-Pathogenesis
  - Macrophage or neutrophil disorder
    - Phagocytic defect often seen with bone marrow suppression, chemotherapy, leukemia, bone marrow transplant
  - B-cell disorder
    - Antibody defect either primary (x-linked agammaglobulinemia or immunoglobulin deficiency) or secondary from multiple myeloma, Waldenstroms, CLL
  - T-cell disorder

Immunocompromised Host

- Cell mediated defect either primary (DiGeorge or Nezelof syndrome) or secondary to AIDS, lymphoma, leukemia, aging
  - Edema
    - Multifactorial: High volumes of fluid for chemotherapy, chemotherapy or radiation damage to heart, minor transfusion reactions, anemia

Gross Pathologic-Surgical Features
- Splenectomy
  - Encapsulated bacteria: Streptococcus, Hemophilus Inf, Staphylococcus
- Mucosal disruption: Candida, gram negative organisms
- Phagocytic dysfunction at risk for
  - Staphlococcus, gram negatives, and aspergillus and mucor
- Antibody dysfunction at risk for
  - Encapsulated bacteria: Staphylococcus, Hemophilus
- Cell mediated dysfunction at risk for
  - Intracellar pathogens, Streptococcus, pseudomonas, mycobacteria, Nocardia, Legionella, cryptococcus, Histoplasmosis, Coccicidimycosis, varicella-zoster, CMV, EBV, PCP, Toxoplasmosis

Microscopic Features
- Even with sampling, a precise cause not identified in 20%

Clinical Issues

Presentation
- Often nonspecific findings, fever may not be due to infection
- Graft vs. Host Disease
  - Acute (donor T cell damage): Skin, liver, GI mucosa primary targets
  - Chronic (autoimmune): Aspects of Sjögrens, SLE, scleroderma esophageal motility, Bronchiolitis obliterans, lichen planus, sicca

Natural History
- Solid organ transplantation
  - < 1 month: aspiration, wound infection, line colonization
  - 1 – 4 months: CMV, PCP, Aspergillus, Nocardia, Mycobacteria
  - > 4 months: Cryptococcus, PCP, Legionella
- BMT
  - < 30 days: Edema pseudomonas, aspiration, hemorrhage
  - 30 – 100 days: CMV, PCP, drugs, radiation, edema, GVHD
  - > 100 days: Streptococcus, Staph, varicella-zoster, GVHD

Treatment
- Empiric therapy with antibiotics often used in immunosuppressed, if no response more aggressive sampling used
- Empiric diuresis often tried to exclude edema

Prognosis
- Depends on underlying condition, and response to therapy
- Establishing a cause by an invasive procedure may not improve outcome by more than 20%

Selected References
1. Logan PM et al: Acute lung disease in the immunocompromised host. Diagnostic accuracy of the chest radiograph. Chest 108:1283-7, 1995
2. Wilson WR et al: Pulmonary disease in the immunocompromised host (2). Mayo Clin Proc 60:610-31, 1985
3. Rosenow EC III et al: Pulmonary disease in the immunocompromised host. Mayo Clin Proc 60:473-87, 1985

AIDS

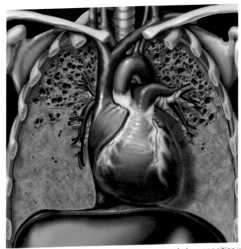

Pneumocystis carinii pneumonia and AIDS. Diffuse ground glass opacities with multiple thin walled pneumatoceles. There is a predilection for the pneumatoceles to occur in the upper lobes.

Key Facts
- Worldwide epidemic to Human Immunodeficiency Virus (HIV)
- 50% develop pulmonary complications: Infections and malignancies
- Nearly 50% pneumonias bacterial
- Non-Hodgkin's Lymphoma most common malignancy, Kaposi's sarcoma on the decline

Imaging Findings
Chest Radiograph
- May be normal in pneumocystis carinii pneumonia (PCP) or mycobacterial infections
- Solitary Pulmonary Nodule (SPN)
  - Lymphoma, usually well defined
  - Lung cancer, kaposi's sarcoma usually ill defined
- Multiple pulmonary nodules
  - PCP, cryptococcus, CMV, nocardia, mycobacteria, lymphoma, metastases
- Cavitating pulmonary nodules
  - Lymphoma, septic emboli, nocardia, mycobacteria, cryptococcus, metastases
- Cysts
  - PCP, lymphocyte interstitial pneumonia (LIP)
- Pleural effusion
  - Kaposi's sarcoma, lymphoma, mycobacteria, bacterial or fungal infection
- Adenopathy
  - Infection (mycobacterial or fungal, bacillary angiomatosis), Kaposi's, lymphoma, thymic hyperplasia
- Central basilar interstitial thickening
  - PCP, Kaposi's, lymphocytic interstitial pneumonia, CMV

AIDS

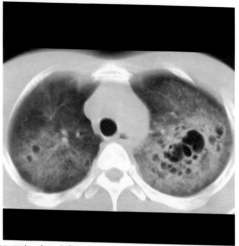

PCP with pneumatoceles. Diffuse ground glass opacities with clusters of thin-walled cystic spaces, predominantly in the upper lobes.

- Focal consolidation
  - Bacterial pneumonia, lymphoma
- PCP (on the decline)
  - May be normal
  - Diffuse central micronodular interstitial thickening
  - Upper lobe cystic disease (10%), predisposed to spontaneous pneumothorax
  - Adenopathy or pleural effusion unusual
- Cryptococcus (most common fungal infection)
  - Diffuse interstitial thickening
  - Pleural fluid
  - Adenopathy
  - Multiple nodules may be cavitated
- Kaposi's sarcoma
  - Nodules (85%), flame-shaped, ill-defined margins, perihilar
  - Interstitial pattern (40%), especially long central linear opacities
  - Adenopathy (50%)
  - Atelectasis, lobar (5%), due to endobronchial Kaposi
- Lymphoma (high-grade B cell non-Hodgkin's)
  - Nodules (20%), well defined, may rapidly enlarge or cavitate
  - Consolidation – interstitial pattern (20%), nonspecific
  - Pleural effusions (50%)
  - Adenopathy (20%)
- Pattern may vary with CD4 count
  - Tuberculosis
    - > 200 cells/mm^3: Post-primary pattern
    - 50–200 cells/mm^3: Primary pattern
    - < 50 cells/mm^3: Military interstitial pattern
    - Paradoxical response: Transient worsening of radiographic pattern with antiviral therapy (strengthened hypersensitivity response)
- Previously irradiated lung protects from PCP

AIDS

<u>CT Findings</u>
- More sensitive than chest radiography, used for selected cases
- Centriacinar nodules < 1 cm usually infectious
- Nodules > 1 cm usually neoplastic
- Peribronchovascular distribution: Kaposi's
- Cavitation or tree-in-bud: Infectious
- Enhancing adenopathy: Mycobacteria
- Amorphous nodal calcification: PCP

<u>Imaging Recommendations</u>
- Chest radiographs usually sufficient for detection and follow-up

Differential Diagnosis
- None

Pathology
<u>General</u>
- HIV infection depletes helper T cells (CD4) leading to immunosuppression
- Typically CD4 count 800-1000 cells/mm^3, HIV depletes 50 cells/year (prodromal period approximately 10 years)
- Epidemiology
  - Spread through close contact with bodily fluids
  - At risk: Multiple sexual partners, IV drug abuse, hemophiliacs

<u>Gross Pathologic-Surgical Features</u>
- LIP may be direct effect of HIV or EB virus on lung
- Pathologic findings not specific to HIV
- PCP normally found in lung, may be either reactivation or reinfection

<u>Microscopic Features</u>
- Infections require sputum or tissue sampling, silver stain for PCP

Clinical Issues
<u>Presentation</u>
- AIDS defining illness, generally occurs when CD4 count < 200 cells/mm^3

<u>Treatment</u>
- Prophylactic treatment for PCP
  - Trimethoprim-sulfamethoxazole (Bactrim)
  - Aerosolized pentamidine
- Antibiotics for specific infections
- Radiation chemotherapy for malignancies
- Retroviral therapy
  - Zidovudine (AZT)
- Viral immunization in the future

<u>Prognosis</u>
- With malignancies, generally poor
- Marked improvement with retroviral therapy

Selected References
1. Kuhlman JE: Pneumocystic infections: The radiologist's perspective. Radiology 198:623-35, 1996
2. Kang EY et al: Detection and differential diagnosis of pulmonary infections and tumors in patients with AIDS: Value of chest radiography versus CT. AJR 166:15-9, 1996

Mycobacterial Infection

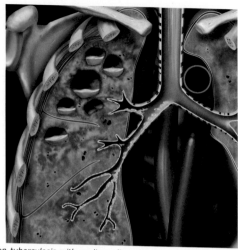

Reactivation tuberculosis with cavitary disease in the apical posterior segments of the upper lobe and superior segment of the lower lobe. Bronchogenic spread to the dependent right lower lobe from spillage of the cavity contents. Apical pleural thickening suggests active granulomatous disease, mycetomas, or tumor.

Key Facts
- Most infected patients have a + purified protein derivative (PPD) and a normal chest radiograph
- Primary tuberculosis (TB): Consolidation, lymphadenopathy and effusion
- Reactivation TB: Cavities in upper dorsal lung (apical-posterior segments)
- The radiographic differential diagnosis includes lung cancer
- Poor response to treatment: Consider AIDS, drug-resistant TB

Imaging Findings
General Features
- Best imaging clue: Fibrocavitary disease in dorsal aspect upper lobes
Chest Radiograph
- Primary TB
  - Most infected patients have a +PPD and a normal chest radiograph
  - Focal consolidation in any lobe, cavitation uncommon (10-30%)
    - Indolent, weeks to months to clear
    - Evolves into a scar, calcified nodule (20%), or clears completely
  - Ipsilateral hilar/mediastinal adenopathy common
  - Pleural effusion (25%): Usually unilateral and small
  - Bronchostenosis, segmental or lobar
  - Primary pneumonia commonly results in a calcified lung nodule (Ghon lesion) and calcified ipsilateral lymph nodes (Ranke complex)
- Reactivation TB
  - Patchy subsegmental consolidation located in apical/posterior segments of upper lobes, superior segments of lower lobes
  - Bilateral, right apex more severe than left apex
  - Cavitation, with or without air fluid levels
  - Pneumothorax uncommon
  - Bronchogenic spread: Intrabronchial spread of cavity contents
  - Endobronchial TB may result in either

Mycobacterial Infection

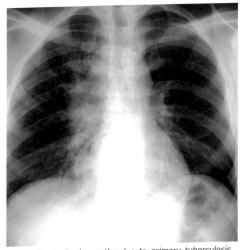

Right hilar and mediastinal adenopathy due to primary tuberculosis. Differential would include bronchogenic carcinoma, lymphoma, or other fungal pneumonia.

- Bronchostenosis causing atelectasis or emphysema
- Bronchiectasis
  - Miliary TB: 2-3 mm nodules may be missed with chest radiography
    - Detected as they increase in size and number
    - Pleural effusion uncommon
  - HIV and TB
    - CD4 count < 200/mm^3, primary TB pattern
    - CD4 count > 200/mm^3, reactivation TB pattern

CT Findings
- May demonstrate findings not appreciated with radiography
  - Bronchogenic spread
  - Peribronchial patchy opacities or centrilobular rosettes
  - Branching nodulation - tree in bud appearance
  - Miliary disease: Profuse uniform distribution of 2-3 mm nodules
  - Lymph nodes: Low density center and peripheral rim enhancement

Complications
- Fibrosing mediastinitis
- Empyema, bronchopleural fistula, burrow into chest wall (empyema necessitatis)
- Pericardial involvement may give rise to constrictive pericarditis
- Hemoptysis may be due to mycetomas, bronchiectasis, or broncholith

Imaging Recommendation
- Chest radiographs usually sufficient for diagnosis and monitoring therapy
- CT useful to detect complications such as mediastinal fibrosis, bronchostenosis and demonstrates important features such as cavitation
  - May be difficult to evaluate for active disease or lung cancer in patients with chronic fibrocavitary disease

Differential Diagnosis
Chronic Fungal Infection
- Histoplasmosis, coccidiomycosis, sporotrochosis

55

Mycobacterial Infection

- Resembles post-primary TB

Ankylosing Spondylitis
- Associated spine changes, TB must be excluded by culture

Progressive Massive Fibrosis (PMF)
- PMF masses may cavitate, usually located in upper lobes
- Appropriate occupational exposure history
- Increased incidence of tuberculosis, TB must be excluded by culture

Sarcoid
- End-stage sarcoid pattern often upper-lobe fibrocavitary disease
- Adenopathy may be absent

Pathology
General
- Caseating granuloma due to mycobacterial infection
- Etiology-Pathogenesis-Pathophysiology
  o Increased susceptibility in patients with impaired cellular immunity
    ▪ HIV positive, elderly, prisoners, indigent and homeless
- Primary TB
  o Delayed hypersensitivity 4-10 weeks after initial exposure, then +PPD
  o Pneumonia with caseous necrosis and regional lymphadenitis
  o Pulmonary focus may evolve into tuberculomas
- Reactivation TB
  o Immediate hypersensitivity
  o Pneumonia, cavity formation
  o Scarring, distortion, bronchiectasis, bronchostenosis, cysts, bullae

Microscopic Features
- Acid-fast bacilli located in macrophages, obligate aerobe

Clinical Issues
Presentation
- Variable: Primary pneumonia often asymptomatic, miliary disease with nonspecific malaise and weight loss

Natural History
- Primary disease self-limited, many years later may develop reactivation

Treatment
- Respiratory isolation for cavitary disease or grossly positive sputum smear until antibiotics instituted
- Anti-tuberculous drugs depending on sensitivity
- Pleural effusion (pleurisy) does not require chest tube drainage, will resolve with antibiotics
- Tuberculous empyema requires chest tube drainage
- Poor response to treatment, consider AIDS or drug-resistant TB
- Bronchial artery embolization or surgery for hemoptysis

Prognosis
- Variable depending on drug resistance and health of host

Selected References
1. Goo JM et al: CT of tuberculosis and nontuberculous mycobacterial infections. Radiol Clin North Am 40(1): 73-87, 2002
2. Saurborn DP et al: The imaging spectrum of pulmonary tuberculosis in AIDS. J Thorac Imaging 17(1):28-33, 2002
3. Kim HY et al: Thoracic sequelae and complications of tuberculosis. Radiographics 21 (4): 839-58, discussion 859-60, 2001

PocketRadiologist™
Chest
Top 100 Diagnoses

AIRWAYS

Tracheobronchomegaly

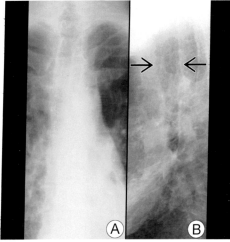

Tracheobronchomegaly. Contour abnormalities of the trachea are often subtle and easily overlooked. (A) The trachea measures 32mm in diameter. On the lateral view (B), the wall is corrigated (arrows).

Key Facts
- Marked dilatation of trachea and major bronchi
- Idiopathic (Mounier-Kuhn), or seen with Ehlers-Danlos syndrome, cutis laxa, and ataxia telangiectasia
- Congenital atrophy or absence of elastic fibers and thinning of smooth muscle layer in trachea and main bronchi
- Recurrent infections may lead to bronchiectasis and pulmonary fibrosis
- Obstructive airways disease from collapse of trachea and major bronchi

Imaging Findings
General Features
- Best imaging clue: Tracheal enlargement > 30 mm diameter
Chest Radiograph
- Marked dilatation of trachea and major bronchi
- Trachea measurements, normal (coronal-sagittal, mm)– men > 25-27; women > 21-23
- Main bronchi, normal (right-left, in mm): men 21, 18.4; women 19.8, 17.4
- Airways dilated on inspiration, collapse on expiration
- Tracheobronchial diverticula
- Bronchiectasis and pulmonary fibrosis, less common
- Hyperinflation
CT Findings
- HRCT more sensitive for bronchiectasis, emphysema, pulmonary fibrosis
Imaging Recommendations
- Chest radiographs usually sufficient for diagnosis, often overlooked
- HRCT for bronchiectasis

Differential Diagnosis
- None, clinical exam to determine cause, i.e., Ehlers-Danlos

Tracheobronchomegaly

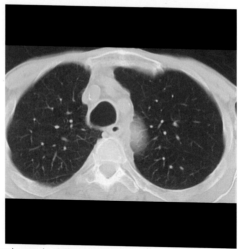

Tracheobronchomegaly. Different patient. Trachea is abnormally dilated but the wall is of normal thickness. Lung is also normal.

Pathology

<u>General</u>
- Atrophy or absence of elastic fibers and thinning of smooth muscle layer in trachea and main bronchi
- Genetics
  - May be congenital or seen with Ehlers-Danlos, cutis laxa, or ataxia telangiectasia
  - Idiopathic dilatation (Mounier-Kuhn) probably also congenital but not known
- Etiology-pathogenesis
  - Loss of elastic or cartilaginous support allows trachea to dilate
- Epidemiology
  - Rare, usually identified in adults, rare in infants or children

<u>Gross Pathologic-Surgical Features</u>
- Enlarged trachea with thinning of the tracheal wall, may contain diverticula

<u>Microscopic Features</u>
- No specific features, absence of elastic fibers, thinning smooth muscle, abnormal cartilage

Clinical Issues

<u>Presentation</u>
- May be asymptomatic
- Loud, productive cough, hoarseness, dyspnea, pneumonia(s)
- Obstructive airway disease from collapse of trachea and major bronchi (tracheomalacia)

<u>Natural History</u>
- Even with congenital cause, symptoms usually don't develop until adulthood, some patients remain asymptomatic

<u>Treatment</u>
- Treated for recurrent infections

Tracheobronchomegaly

- Pneumococcal immunization

Prognosis
- Depends on the development of obstructive airways disease

Selected References
1. Woodring et al: Acquired tracheomegaly in adults as a complication of diffuse pulmonary fibrosis. AJR 152: 743-7, 1989
2. Katz I et al: Tracheobronchomegaly: Mounier-Kuhn syndrome. AJR 88: 1084-94, 1962

Dyskinetic Cilia Syndrome

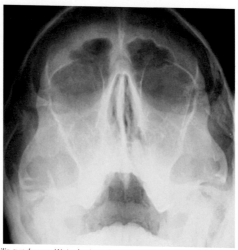

Dysmotile cilia syndrome. Water's view. Complete opacification of the maxillary sinuses.

Key Facts
- Synonym: Kartagener syndrome
- Triad: Situs inversus or dextrocardia, sinusitis, bronchiectasis
- Dyskinetic cilia and/or spermatozoa
- Recurrent sinus, ear and pulmonary infections, male infertility
- Functional and/or structural abnormalities of cilia and spermatozoa

Imaging Findings
General Features
- Best imaging clue: Bronchiectasis and dextrocardia
Chest Radiograph
- Situs inversus (50%) or dextrocardia in patient or sibling, paranasal sinusitis, bronchiectasis
- Other associated abnormalities: Transposition of the great vessels, trilocular or bilocular heart, pyloric stenosis, hypospadias, post-cricoid web (Paterson-Brown-Kelly syndrome)
- Bronchial wall thickening, hyperinflation, segmental atelectasis, consolidation, segmental bronchiectasis (often lower lobes)
CT Findings
- HRCT more sensitive for bronchiectasis and recurrent pneumonias involving mostly lower lobes and right middle lobe
Imaging Recommendations
- Chest radiography usually sufficient for diagnosis, HRCT may be useful to determine presence and extent of bronchiectasis

Differential Diagnosis
- None

Pathology
General
- Genetics

Dyskinetic Cilia Syndrome

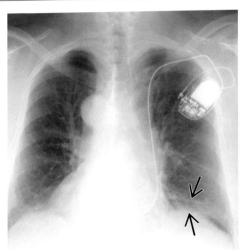

Karteganers. Situs inversus. Linear tramtracking in both lower lobes consistent with bronchiectasis (arrows).

- o Autosomal recessive, 1 in 20,000, males = females
- Etiology-pathogenesis
  - o Uncoordinated and ineffective motion of cilia and/or spermatozoa
  - o Lack of ciliary motion results in dextrocardia (no in utero cardiac rotation)
  - o Lack of clearance of airway secretions results in recurrent infections and eventual bronchiectasis

Gross Pathologic-Surgical Features
- Dextrocardia or situs inversus
- Diffuse bronchiectasis

Microscopic Features
- Cilia normally have 2 central microtubules connected by radial spokes to 9 outer doublet microtubules
- In dyskinetic cilia syndrome, the outer microtubules lack dynein arms, can be demonstrated by electron microscopy

Clinical Issues

Presentation
- Chronic rhinitis, sinusitis, otitis, recurrent bronchitis, bronchiectasis, pneumonias, small airways disease, corneal abnormalities, poor sense of smell
- Absent or reduced tracheobronchial mucociliary clearance
- Defective neutrophil chemotaxis
- Characteristic ultrastructural defects of nasal or bronchial cilia
- Immotile spermatozoa, infertile males
- Females are fertile

Natural History
- Airways normal at birth, abnormal ciliary function eventually results in stasis of secretions in airways, recurrent infections and bronchiectasis

Treatment
- Rotating antibiotics for bronchiectasis

Dyskinetic Cilia Syndrome

- Postural drainage
- Genetic counseling

Prognosis
- Disability due to severity of bronchiectasis

Selected References
1. Nadel HR et al: The immotile cilia syndrome: Radiological manifestations. Radiology 154:651-5, 1985
2. Eliasson R et al: The immotile-cilia syndrome. A congenital ciliary abnormality as an etiologic factor in chronic airway infections and male sterility. N Engl J Med 297:1-6, 1977

Tracheopathia Osteoplastica

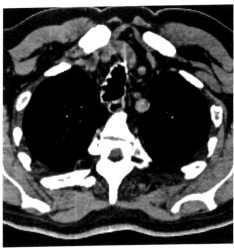

Multiple calcified nodules along the lateral wall of the trachea. Patient was asymptomatic. Tracheopathia osteochondroplastica.

Key Facts
- Nodularity or undulating thickening of tracheal cartilaginous rings and bronchi
- Nodules may be calcified
- Diagnosis made at bronchoscopy or with CT
- Enchondroses of cartilage rings
- Rare
- Usually asymptomatic

Imaging Findings
General Features
- Best imaging clue: Small nodules anterolateral tracheal cartilaginous rings
Chest Radiograph
- Nodularity or undulating thickening of trachea and bronchi
- Most have normal chest radiograph
- Calcification of nodules usually not evident on radiograph
- Large nodules may cause recurrent pneumonias or atelectasis
CT Findings
- CT more sensitive, examination of choice
- Nodular thickening of anterior and lateral walls of trachea
- Involves lower two-thirds of trachea and main segmental and lobar bronchi
- Spares posterior tracheal membrane (no cartilage)
- Rarely produce airway narrowing or atelectasis
- Nodules calcified at CT
Imaging Recommendations
- Usually incidental finding identified at CT

Tracheopathia Osteoplastica

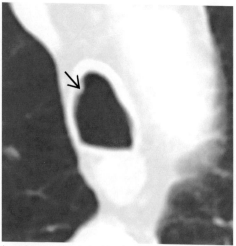

Non-calcified nodule along the anterior lateral wall of the trachea (arrow). The posterior wall is spared due to lack of cartilage.

Differential Diagnosis:

Amyloid
- Calcified nodules involve posterior tracheal membrane in addition to the anterior and lateral walls

Laryngeal Papillomatosis
- Nodules don't calcify
- Younger patients
- May have multiple cystic lesions in lung

Wegener's Granulomatosis
- Diffuse nodular thickening of tracheal wall
- Nodules don't calcify
- Often associated with multiple thick-walled pulmonary cavities

Endobronchial Sarcoid
- Nodules rarely calcify
- Nodular bronchovascular thickening within lung not seen with tracheobroncheopathia
- Hilar adenopathy not seen with tracheobroncheopathia

Pathology

General
- Enchondroses and bony nodules of cartilage rings
- Etiology-pathogenesis
  - Unknown cause, may be due to amyloidosis
- Epidemiology
  - Mostly in men, usually > 50 years old

Gross Pathologic-Surgical Features
- Beaded appearance of trachea and bronchi with intact mucosa

Microscopic Features
- Nodules or spicules of cartilage and bone in the submucosa of the trachea and bronchi

Tracheopathia Osteoplastica

Clinical Issues

<u>Presentation</u>
- Most patients are asymptomatic
- Occasionally dyspnea, hoarseness, cough, expectoration, wheezing, hemoptysis, recurrent pneumonias
- Diagnosis made at bronchoscopy or with CT

<u>Natural History</u>
- Progresses very slowly

<u>Treatment</u>
- Endoscopic therapy or surgery for obstructing lesions

<u>Prognosis</u>
- Excellent
- Death from airway obstruction, rare

Selected References
1. Onitsuka H et al: Computed tomography of tracheopathia osteoplastica. AJR 140:268-70, 1983
2. Young RH et al: Tracheopathia osteoplastica: Clinical, radiologic, and pathological correlations. J Thorac Cardiovasc Surg 79:537-41, 1980

Tracheal Stenosis

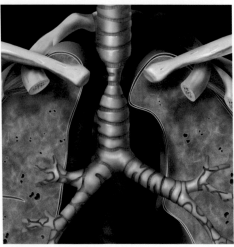

Circumferential tracheal stenosis at the thoracic inlet. This may occur following prolonged intubation.

Key Facts
- Coronal and sagittal diameters < 13 mm in men and 10 mm in women
- Expiratory CT will show if lesion is fixed or due to tracheomalacia
- Spiral CT with thin cuts and multiplanar or 3-D reconstructions best to define lesion(s)
- Intubation or tracheostomy, very common cause of stenosis
- Patients may be misdiagnosed as having asthma
- Asymptomatic until tracheal diameter decreased 50%

Imaging Findings
General Features
- Best imaging clue: Tracheal pathology commonly overlooked, "blind spot"
Chest Radiograph
- Coronal and sagittal diameters < 13 mm in men and 10 mm in women
- Post intubation – stenosis typically above thoracic inlet, concentric and may be long, short or involve multiple segments
- Post tracheostomy – at level of stoma, inflatable cuff, or 1–1.5 cm distal to inferior margin of tip of tube; circumferential narrowing approx 2 cm long, thin, cross-sectional web, or eccentric soft-tissue density
- Tumor: Intraluminal nodules, smooth, irregular or lobulated
CT Findings
- Inspiratory and expiratory CT will show if the lesion is fixed
- Spiral CT with thin sections (3 mm collimation)
- Multiplanar and 3-D reconstructions will show anatomy in complex lesions
- Malignant tumors can be focal, circumferential, sessile or polypoid; most from 2 to 4 cm
- Benign tumors do not extend beyond the tracheal wall
Imaging Recommendations
- CT to define anatomy and relationship to surrounding mediastinal structures

Tracheal Stenosis

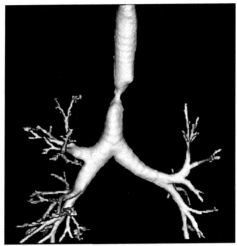

3-D reconstruction of focal tracheal stenosis secondary to intubation.

Differential Diagnosis

<u>None</u>
<u>Associated Causes Include</u>
- Traumatic – intubation, tracheostomy, trauma
- Extrinsic – e.g., thyroid goiter, lymphadenopathy/mass, fibrosing mediastinitis, vascular ring
- Intrinsic – benign and malignant tumors, lymphoma, extension of mediastinal tumor, metastases
- Infection – croup, papillomatosis, TB, bacillary angiomatosis, scleroma, fungal
- Immunologic – amyloid, relapsing polychondritis
- Granulomatous – Wegener's granulomatosis, ulcerative colitis, sarcoid
- Idiopathic

Pathology

<u>General</u>
- Trachea uncommon location for malignancies even though exposure to cigarette smoke the same as the lung

<u>Gross Pathologic-Surgical Features</u>
- Traumatic – granulation tissue and fibrosis of mucosa lining the tracheal cartilage rings
- Neoplasms
  - o Malignant tumors: Rare, usually squamous cell, mostly in men
  - o Adenoid cystic carcinoma, less common, males = females
  - o Lymphoma, chloroma
  - o Benign tumors: Rare, neurogenic tumors, leiomyomas

<u>Microscopic Features</u>
- Specific to neoplastic or benign pathology

Tracheal Stenosis

Clinical Issues

Presentation
- Hoarseness, cough, wheeze, stridor and dyspnea with exertion
- If x-ray requisition states asthma, look for tracheal stenosis
- Rarely, hypoventilation, hypoxemia, hypercarbia, pulmonary artery hypertension, cor pulmonale
- Inspiratory wheeze if lesion extrathoracic; expiratory wheeze if lesion intrathoracic
- Post intubation - symptoms may appear several weeks to years after intubation

Natural History
- Stenosis often overlooked for years, patients treated for "asthma"

Treatment
- Tracheal stenosis due to fibrosis and benign tumors may be amenable to surgical correction
- Malignancies usually advanced at diagnosis

Prognosis
- Malignant tracheal tumors have very poor prognosis

Selected References
1.   Marom EM et al: Focal abnormalities of the trachea and main bronchi. AJR 176: 707-11, 2001
2.   Breatnach E et al: Dimensions of the normal human trachea. AJR 142:903-6, 1984

Amyloidosis

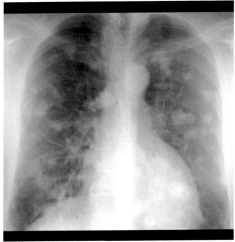

Primary pulmonary amyloid. Multiple pulmonary nodules contain several foci of calcification. Heart mildly enlarged.

Key Facts
- Primary or secondary to chronic malignancies or inflammatory disease
- 10% of patients with multiple myeloma develop amyloidosis
- Bleeding common due to amyloid deposition in vessels
- Tracheobronchial > pulmonary nodular > adenopathy > diffuse septal
- Calcification more common in localized deposits

Imaging Findings
General Features
- Best imaging clue: Multiple calcified tracheal or pulmonary nodules
Chest Radiograph
- Tracheobronchial
  - Nodular deposits more common than diffuse thickening
  - Subglottic location most common
  - 30% calcify
- Pulmonary nodular
  - Equally divided between single or multiple
  - 20% calcify, growth very slow
  - Sharply-marginated, peripheral, lobulated, variable-sized nodule(s)
  - Midlung, right lung 2x left lung
  - Cavitation extremely rare; not associated with adenopathy
- Adenopathy
  - Usually multiple lymph node groups involved
  - May be massive
  - Stippled, diffuse or even eggshell calcification
  - Often combined with diffuse interstitial thickening
- Diffuse septal
  - Miliary nodules
  - Peripheral basilar septal thickening and honeycombing
- Other
  - Cardiac enlargement due to amyloid deposition

Amyloidosis

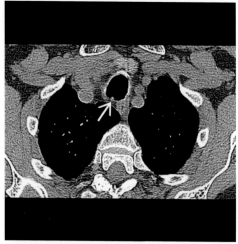

Tracheal amyloid. Calcified nodule in posterior tracheal membrane. (Arrow) tracheopathia osteochondroplastica arises from cartilage and would not arise from the posterior tracheal membrane.

- o Pleural effusions rare, usually associated with cardiac disease
- o Soft-tissue deposition

CT Findings
- More sensitive then chest radiograph, more sensitive for calcification
- Diffuse pulmonary disease usually associated with adenopathy

Imaging Recommendations
- CT useful to characterize lung and tracheal lesions for distribution and presence of calcification

Differential Diagnosis
Tracheobronchial Amyloid
- Primary benign and malignant tumors
  - o Usually focal, not diffuse
- Tracheopathia osteochondroplastica
  - o Nodules located only along anterior and lateral walls
  - o Amyloid circumferential
- Relapsing polychondritis
  - o No nodules
  - o Clinical findings in sclerae or ears
- Rhinoscleroma
  - o Paranasal sinus disease
  - o Culture for Klebsiella

Nodular
- Differential for solitary pulmonary nodule (SPN) and multiple pulmonary nodules including primary carcinoma, metastases, granulomatosis disease, benign metastasizing leiomyomas, rheumatoid arthritis

Adenopathy
- Lymphoma: Does not calcify prior to treatment
- Sarcoid
  - o Symmetrical enlargement

Amyloidosis

   - o Often associated peribronchial interstitial lung disease
- Tuberculosis: Nodes often have rim enhancement
- Metastases: Not likely to calcify (unless from bone or chondroid tumor)

Diffuse Septal
- Differential for interstitial lung disease including usual interstitial pneumonia (UIP), scleroderma, rheumatoid arthritis, BOOP, drug toxicity

Pathology
General
- Extracellular protein deposition
- Vascular deposition leads to fragility and bleeding

Microscopic Features
- Birefringent apple-green fluorescence under polarized light with Congo red stain
- Large sheets of protein deposition

Clinical Issues
Presentation
- Usually asymptomatic
  - o Tracheobronchial: Cough, wheezing, hemoptysis
  - o Diffuse septal: Dyspnea
- Tracheobronchial: Male 2:1, average age 50
- Nodular: No gender prevalence, average age 65
- Diffuse septal: No gender prevalence, average age 55
- Primary or myeloma associated (AL type protein)
  - o Most patients with amyloid have monoclonal spike
  - o Conversely <25% with monoclonal gammopathy develop amyloidosis
  - o 10% of patients with multiple myeloma develop amyloidosis
  - o Other organs involved: Heart, kidney, tongue, GI tract, skin, muscle
- Secondary (AA type)
  - o Inflammation: RA, bronchiectasis, CF, osteomyelitis, Crohn's
  - o Malignancies: Renal cell, medullary thyroid carcinoma, Hodgkin's
  - o Familial (AF type) also with Mediterranean fever
  - o Senile (AS type)
    - ▪ Generally asymptomatic, common (90% over 90 years of age)
    - ▪ Associated with cardiac deposition

Treatment
- Resection to alleviate symptoms in tracheobronchial obstruction
  - o Often recurs
- No known treatment for diffuse forms, supportive therapy only

Prognosis
- Prognosis poor for diffuse disease (survival < 2 years)

Selected References
1. Pickford HA et al: Thoracic cross-sectional imaging of amyloidosis. AJR 168:351-5, 1997
2. Stark P et al: Manifestations of esophageal disease on plain chest radiographs. AJR 155:729-34, 1990
3. Gedgaudas-Mcclees et al: Thoracic findings in gastrointestinal pathology. Radiol Clin North Am 22:563-89, 1984

Bronchiectasis

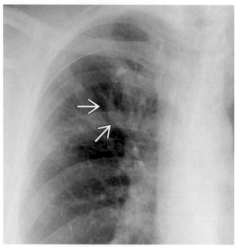

Alergic bronchopulmonary aspergillosis (ABPA). Bronchiectasis right upper lobe. Mucoid-filled bronchi have "finger in glove" appearance (arrows).

Key Facts
- Chronic, irreversible dilatation of bronchi
- Severity: Saccular > varicose > cylindrical
- Radiography shows tram lines, ring shadows, crowded bronchial markings, long bands
- HRCT shows dilated bronchi, thickened bronchial walls, signet ring sign, air trapping, mosaic pattern, volume loss
- Many other associated diseases should be considered
- Important cause of hemoptysis, sometimes massive

Imaging Findings
General Features
- Best imaging clue: Tram lines and ring shadows

Chest Radiograph
- Tram lines – parallel thickened lines representing the thickened bronchial walls
- Ring or curvilinear opacities, 5 to 20 mm
- Band shadows – fluid or mucous-filled bronchi, they may branch and point to hilum
- Hyperinflation or atelectasis indicated by vascular crowding, displaced fissures
- Dilated bronchi may be cylindrical, varicose, or saccular (mild to severe)
- Scarring, bullae, pleural thickening
- Central bronchiectasis
  - Allergic bronchopulmonary aspergillosis
    - Asthmatics and cystic fibrosis at risk
    - Fleeting subsegmental consolidation
    - Primarily upper lobes
    - "Finger in glove" appearance from impacted central bronchi

Bronchiectasis

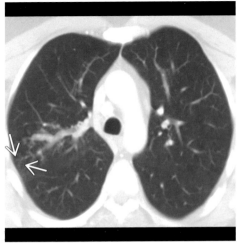

CT ABPA. Bronchiectasis right upper lobe. Bronchus is mucoid filled. Distally centrilobular nodules represent mucoid-filled small airways (arrows).

<u>CT Findings</u>
- HRCT - best imaging modality for detection of bronchial wall thickening and dilatation
- Normal bronchus same size or smaller than adjacent artery
  - "Signet ring sign" bronchus larger than adjacent artery
  - Normal bronchi may be larger than artery at altitude
- Bronchial wall thickening
- Abnormal bronchial tapering
- Cylindrical, varicose or saccular
- May have air-fluid levels
- Expiration HRCT will show associated small airway disease or obliterative bronchiolitis indicated by air trapping and a more pronounced "mosaic pattern"
- Secretions within peripheral small, centrilobular bronchioles can give V- or Y- shaped opacities – "tree-in-bud"
- Volume loss, subtle or segmental or lobar
- Advanced cases may be difficult to distinguish from fibrosis with honeycombing

<u>Imaging Recommendation</u>
- HRCT for diagnosis and characterization of severity and extent

Differential Diagnosis
<u>Atelectasis or Pneumonia</u>
- May have bronchial dilatation that is reversible
- Wait 3 months after infection resolved and re-image

<u>Normal</u>
- Bronchi may be slightly dilated at altitude due to hypoxic vasodilatation

Pathology
<u>General</u>
- Chronic, local, irreversible dilatation of bronchi

Bronchiectasis

- Embryology
  - Dyskinetic cilia syndrome (Kartagener's): Situs inversus, dextrocardia congenital defect in cilia, bronchiectasis acquired because of lack of cilia action in host defense
- Etiology-pathogenesis
  - Post-infection (TB, mycobacterium avium intracellulare (MAI), fungal, bacterial, viral)
  - Cystic fibrosis
  - Swyer-James syndrome
  - Chronic aspiration
  - Toxic inhalation
  - Rheumatoid arthritis
  - Combined immunodeficiency syndrome
  - Allergic bronchopulmonary aspergillosis (ABPA)
  - Panbronchiolitis
  - Mounier-Kuhn syndrome
  - Congenital

Gross Pathologic-Surgical Features
- Bronchial walls thickened and chronically inflamed with granulation tissue and fibrosis
- Bronchial artery hypertrophy
- Leads to bronchial wall weakness, recurrent infections, parenchymal volume loss and distortion

Microscopic Features
- No specific features, chronic inflammation to both airway wall and lung, fibrosis

Clinical Issues

Presentation
- Onset, often in childhood, post pertussis or severe bacterial pneumonia
- Incidence decreased with immunization and liberal use of antibiotics
- With mild disease, may be asymptomatic
- Cough, dyspnea, copious purulent sputum, recurrent infections, cor pulmonale
- Hemoptysis, sometimes massive
- Good's syndrome: Bronchiectasis, hypogammaglobulinemia, thymoma

Treatment
- Surgery for localized disease
- Bronchial artery embolization to control hemoptysis

Prognosis
- Depends on severity

Selected References
1. McGuinness G et al: Bronchiectasis: CT evaluation. AJR 160 253-9, 1993
2. Grenier P et al: Bronchiectasis: Assessment by thin-section CT. Radiology 161:95-9, 1986

Cystic Fibrosis

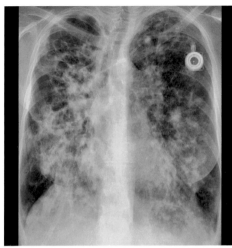

Cystic fibrosis. Severe bronchiectasis and mucus plugging. Lungs are markedly hyperinflated.

Key Facts
- Autosomal recessive gene regulating chloride transport
- Hyperinflation initial manifestation
- Most severe in upper lung zones
- Other common findings, apical cystic airspaces and lobar atelectasis
- Predisposition to spontaneous pneumothorax

Imaging Findings
General Features
- Predominately upper lobe bronchiectasis and mucous plugging
Chest Radiograph
- Initial
  - Hyperinflation
  - Lobar atelectasis, especially right upper lobe
- Later
  - Bronchiectasis
  - Multiple small, ill-defined opacities in lung periphery from small airways mucoid impaction
  - Pneumonia (recurrent)
  - Hilar enlargement
    - Adenopathy from chronic inflammation
    - Cor pulmonale
- Parenchymal changes usually worse in the upper lung zones
- Apical cystic airspaces
- Predisposed to spontaneous pneumothorax
- 10% develop allergic bronchopulmonary aspergillosis (ABPA)
- Brasfield scoring system used clinically
CT Findings
- HRCT: Best imaging modality for detection of bronchial wall thickening and dilatation

Cystic Fibrosis

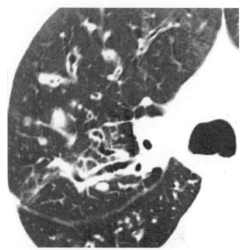

Cystic fibrosis. Bronchiectasis right upper lobe. Typically the degree of bronchiectasis is more severe in the upper lobes.

- Normal bronchus same size or smaller than adjacent artery
  - "Signet ring sign" bronchus larger than adjacent artery
  - Normal bronchi may be larger than artery at altitude
- Bronchial wall thickening
- Abnormal bronchial tapering
- Cylindrical, varicose and saccular (in order of severity)
- May have air-fluid levels
- Expiration HRCT will show associated small airway disease or obliterative bronchiolitis indicated by air trapping and a more pronounced "mosaic pattern"
- Secretions within peripheral small centrilobular bronchioles can give V-or Y-shaped opacities – "tree-in-bud"
- Volume loss, subtle or segmental or lobar
- Advanced cases may be difficult to distinguish from fibrosis with honeycombing

Imaging Recommendations
- HRCT to detect bronchiectasis
- Chest radiographs usually sufficient for long-term follow-up

Differential Diagnosis
ABPA
- Central bronchiectasis
- History of asthma, often eosinophilia

Pathology
General
- Lungs normal at birth
- Airways colonized with Pseudomonas
- Genetics
  - Autosomal recessive, Caucasians

Cystic Fibrosis

- o Gene defect that regulates chloride transport across cell membrane
- Etiology-pathogenesis
  - o Pathologic changes acquired from abnormal chloride transport
  - o Abnormal chloride transport produces thick, viscous mucus
  - o Mucus not expectorated, becomes secondarily infected
  - o Repeated infections eventually destroy airways
  - o Increased respiratory excursions in lower lobes aids removal of secretions, thus upper lobe airways predominately affected

Gross Pathologic-Surgical Features
- Bronchial walls thickened and chronically inflamed with granulation tissue and fibrosis
- Bronchial artery hypertrophy
- Leads to bronchial wall weakness, recurrent infections, parenchymal volume loss and distortion
- Colonization with Pseudomonas

Microscopic Features
- No specific features, chronic inflammation both to airway wall and lung

Clinical Issues
Presentation
- Onset in childhood
  - o Meconium ileus at birth – 15%
  - o Failure to thrive
  - o Recurrent respiratory infections
- Diagnosis: Sweat chloride
- With mild disease, may be asymptomatic
- Cough, dyspnea, copious purulent sputum, recurrent infections, cor pulmonale
- Hemoptysis, sometimes massive
- Systemic manifestations
  - o Pancreatic insufficiency
  - o Pansinusitis
  - o Biliary cirrhosis

Treatment
- Pancreatic enzymes
- Respiratory therapy
  - o Postural drainage
  - o Bronchodilators
  - o Prophylactic antibiotics
  - o Aerosolized rh DNase
  - o Lung transplants for endstage disease
  - o Hemoptysis may require bronchial artery embolization
- Gene therapy promising

Prognosis
- Improved but life span shortened
- Death due to cor pulmonale or hemoptysis

Selected References
1. Wood BP: Cystic fibrosis. Radiology 204:1-10, 1997
2. Friedman PJ et al: Pulmonary cystic fibrosis in the adult: Early and late radiologic findings with pathologic correlations. AJR 136: 1131-44, 1981

Bronchial Atresia

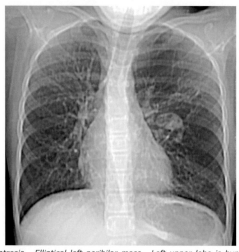

Bronchial atresia. Elliptical left perihilar mass. Left upper lobe is hyperlucent as compared to the right upper lobe.

Key Facts
- Congenital atresia proximal segmental bronchus, normal distal architecture
- Apicoposterior segment left upper lobe most common location
- Suprahilar nodule, upper lobe hyperexpanded and lucent
- Fluid filled at birth

Imaging Findings
Chest Radiograph
- Best imaging clue: Round, sharply-defined, suprahilar mass with distal hyperinflation
- Dilatation and mucoid impaction distal to segmental bronchus
- Round or ovoid mass adjacent to the hilum (bronchocele)
- Neonates; lobe or segment may be fluid filled, gradually replaced by air
- Distal lung hyperinflated
- Most common location: Apicoposterior segment left upper lobe, followed by right upper lobe, right middle lobe; lower lobe bronchi rare

Obstetric Ultrasound
- Can be detected in utero
- Fluid-filled upper lobe
  - Differential
    - Cystic adenomatoid malformation
    - Congenital diaphragmatic hernia
    - Bronchopulmonary foregut malformations
    - Lobar emphysema

Imaging Recommendations
- CT may be useful to characterize bronchial anatomy and characterize nodule

Bronchial Atresia

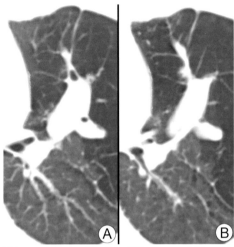

Sequential CT images left upper lobe (A and B). Segemental bronchi to left upper lobe are distended with mucous. Left upper lobe is markedly hyperinflated.

Differential Diagnosis
Congenital Lobar Emphysema
- No mass

Solitary Pulmonary Nodule (SPN)
- No hyperinflation distal to nodule

Allergic Bronchopulmonary Aspergillosis (ABPA)
- Central bronchiectasis
- Bilateral

Cystic Fibrosis
- Bronchiectasis
- Bilateral

Carcinoid Tumor, Slow Growing Endobronchial Tumor
- Mass not as large as mucoid impaction
- Distal lung usually not hyperexpanded but atelectatic

Pathology
General
- Obliteration proximal lumen segmental bronchus
- Aeration distal lung through collateral air drift
- Distal lung: Normal architecture
- Embryology-anatomy
  - Thought to occur between 5th and 15th week of gestation

Gross Pathologic-Surgical Features
- Mucoid-filled lung-forming mass distal to atretic bronchus
- Distal lung hyperinflated but otherwise normal

Microscopic Features
- No specific features, nonspecific inflammation distal to atresia

Clinical Issues
Presentation
- Often asymptomatic, may not come to attention until adulthood

Bronchial Atresia

- May have history of recurrent infections
- Associated with other congenital anomalies
  o Congenital lobar emphysema

<u>Treatment</u>
- Surgical resection

<u>Prognosis</u>
- Excellent

Selected References
1. Keslar P et al: Radiographic manifestation of anomalies of the lung. Radiol Clin North Am 29: 255-70, 1991
2. Simon G et al: Atresia of an apical bronchus of the left upper lobe: Report of 3 cases. Br J Dis Chest 57: 126-32, 1963

Small Airways Disease

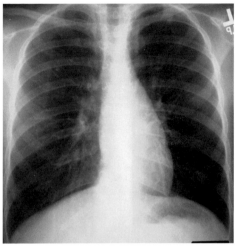

Bronchiolitis obliterans. Progressive shortness of breath (SOB) and dyspnea 14 months following allogeneic bone marrow transplant. Lungs slightly hyperinflated, but otherwise normal.

Key Facts
- Causes include transplants, post viral infection, toxic fume inhalation
- Obstructive hyperinflation, must be severe before PFTs deteriorate
- Swyer-James syndrome special case (unilateral hyperlucent lung)
- HRCT: Mosaic perfusion, mild cylindrical bronchiectasis, centrilobular nodules
- Respiratory bronchiolitis mostly due to smoking

Imaging Findings
General Features
- Best imaging clue: Mosaic perfusion due to hyperinflation

Chest Radiograph
- Usually normal or hyperinflation
- Swyer-James syndrome
  - Unilateral small hyperlucent lung
- Respiratory bronchiolitis: Normal radiograph
- Respiratory bronchiolitis-interstitial lung disease (RB-ILD) mild interstitial thickening

CT Findings
- Mosaic perfusion
  - Lucent lung, small vessels in lucent lung
    - Due to hypoxic vasoconstriction
  - Normal lung (which is of increased attenuation) vessels normal to slightly enlarged
  - Expiratory scanning useful to differentiate from vascular disease
    - Hyperlucent lung will not change, normal lung will increase in attenuation
- Mild cylindrical bronchiectasis and bronchial wall thickening of segmental and subsegmental bronchi
- Occasional centrilobular nodules (rarely tree-in-bud)

Small Airways Disease

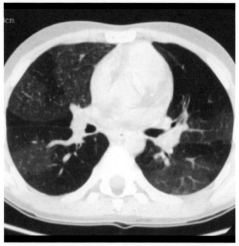

Bronchiolitis obliterans HRCT. Mosaic perfusion pattern is nearly equally divided between ground glass/hypoattenuated areas. In hypoattenuated areas, vessels are extremely small due to hypoxic vasoconstriction. Expiratory scan (not shown) hypoattenuated areas would not increase in density.

Imaging Recommendations
- HRCT, inspiration and expiration to detect air trapping

Differential Diagnosis
Asthma
- No micronodules, mosaic perfusion identical
Panlobular Emphysema
- HRCT changes of emphysema, predominantly lower lobes
Langerhans Cell Granulomatosis
- Micronodules more profuse, cysts, predominantly upper lobes
Desquamative Interstitial Pneumonia (DIP)
- Diffuse ground-glass opacities, usually subpleural or patchy
- Not bronchocentric like RB-ILD
Hypersensitivity Pneumonitis
- Identical radiographic findings
- Chronic disease will have more fibrosis

Pathology
General
- Insult to the small airways (respiratory bronchioles)
- Air flows rapidly down conducting airways (trachea to terminal bronchioles) and then velocity decreases rapidly to allow gas exchange
- Small particles (< 5 microns) escape impacting into larger airways and are deposited on the nonconducting airways (respiratory bronchioles)
  o Causes of constrictive bronchiolitis
    ▪ Idiopathic
    ▪ Toxic fume inhalation (especially silo-filler's disease)

- Post viral or mycoplasma pneumonia: Swyer-James thought to be due to childhood infection
- Chronic allograft rejection: Bone marrow transplants, lung transplants
- Connective tissue disease: Rheumatoid arthritis, systemic lupus erythematosus
- Drugs: Penicillamine

Gross Pathologic-Surgical Features
- Respiratory bronchioles plugged with granulation tissue or fibrous tissue
- Bronchioles concentrically narrowed

Microscopic Features
- Depends on cause
- Respiratory bronchiolitis
  - Pigmented macrophages clustered around respiratory bronchioles
  - When severe: Fibrous scarring into surrounding alveolar walls
  - Seen within 2 years of onset of smoking
- Neuroendocrine cell hyperplasia
- Follicular hyperplasia
- Extrinsic allergic alveolitis
  - Poorly-formed granulomas

Clinical Issues

Presentation
- Idiopathic bronchiolitis obliterans usually seen in females 40-60 years of age
- Cough, dyspnea
- Respiratory bronchiolitis: Asymptomatic, if symptomatic known as RB-ILD
- Respiratory bronchiolitis not specific to smoking, seen in other dust exposures
- Respiratory bronchiolitis may be precursor of centriacinar emphysema

Treatment
- Smoking cessation or removal from dusty environment
- Steroids for RB-ILD

Prognosis
- Little known about natural history, some suggestion that respiratory bronchiolitis is precursor of centriacinar emphysema

Selected References
1. Desai SR et al: Small airways disease: Expiratory computed tomography comes of age. Clin Radiol 52:332-7, 1997
2. Garg K et al: Proliferative and constrictive bronchiolitis: Classification and radiologic features. AJR 162:803-8, 1994
3. McLoud TC et al: Bronchiolitis obliterans. Radiology 159:1-8, 1986

PocketRadiologist™
Chest
Top 100 Diagnoses

INTERSTITIAL

Sarcoidosis

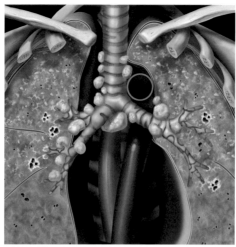

Upper and mid lung diffuse reticulonodular opacities. Symmetrical paratracheal, hilar and subcarinal adenopathy, bronchovascular bundle thickening and absence of pleural disease are very characteristic of sarcoidosis.

Key Facts
- Common systemic disease of unknown etiology
- Widespread noncaseating granulomas that resolve or cause fibrosis
- May have associated erythema nodosum, uveitis, hypercalcemia, arthritis
- 95% of patients have abnormal chest radiograph with lymphadenopathy and/or lung opacities
- HRCT centriacinar nodules along bronchovascular bundles, septa, and periphery of lobule
- Definitive diagnosis with transbronchial, lymph node, or liver biopsy
- Most patients have a good prognosis with resolution in < 2 years
- Major complications include respiratory failure from fibrosis, mycetomas, hemorrhage, and cor pulmonale

Imaging Findings
General Features
- Best imaging clue: Symmetric hilar adenopathy with nodular interstitial lung disease
Chest Radiograph
- Abnormal chest radiograph – 95%
- 5 to 15% have normal chest radiograph at onset
- Lymphadenopathy
  - (80%) most common finding – bilateral hilar/paratracheal
  - Usually not visible at 2 years; however may persist for many years
  - Nodes may calcify, sometimes eggshell calcification
  - Lung disease (< 50%), often worsens with nodal regression
- Pulmonary
  - Reticulonodular opacities (90%) predominately upper lung zones
  - Large airspace nodules with air bronchograms (alveolar sarcoid)
  - Chronically: Fibrosis mid and upper lung zones

Sarcoidosis

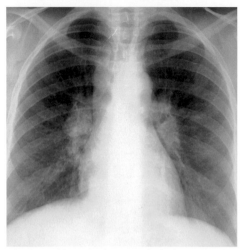

Sarcoidosis. Symmetric hilar and right paratracheal adenopathy. Key is symmetry of enlargement. Differential would include lymphoma, metastases, other granulomatous disease and angioimmunoblastic lymphadenopathy.

- Upper lobe cyst formation (at risk for aspergilloma)
- Atypical appearances
  - Atypical lymphadenopathy - unilateral hilar, posterior mediastinal
  - Unilateral lung disease, cavitary lung lesions, or pleural effusion

CT Findings
- More sensitive than chest radiography for pulmonary disease
- CT nodes also present in left paratracheal, AP window, anterior mediastinum, retroperitoneal lymph node groups
- Pattern: 1-5 mm centrilobular nodules along bronchovascular structures, septa, and periphery of lobule
- Often extends in a swath from the hilum to lung periphery
- Ground-glass opacities, nodular or lobular in size may precede or coexist with nodules
- Progressive massive fibrosis, distortion, honeycombing, cysts, bullae, traction bronchiectasis with chronic severe disease
- Secondary mycetomas in cavities and cysts
- Large and small airway stenoses

Imaging Recommendations
- HRCT useful to characterize interstitial lung disease, chest radiographs usually sufficient for diagnosis

Differential Diagnosis

Berylliosis
- Identical findings, need occupational history

Hypersensitivity Pneumonitis
- No adenopathy, lacks peribronchial distribution

Eosinophilic Granuloma
- Minimal adenopathy, lacks peribronchial distribution

Silicosis
- Occupational history otherwise identical radiographic findings

Sarcoidosis

Lymphoma
- Asymmetric nodal enlargement

Mediastinal Granuloma – Histoplasmosis, TB
- Asymmetric nodal enlargement

Pathology
General
- Widespread noncaseating granulomas that resolve or cause fibrosis
- Etiology-pathogenesis
  - Unknown, sarcoid may follow treatment of lymphoma
- Epidemiology
  - 10 times more common in blacks, female predominance

Gross Pathologic-Surgical Features
- Symmetrically enlarged lymph nodes
- Honeycombing usually more severe in upper lung zones

Microscopic Features
- Well-formed granulomas; central epithelioid histiocytes and multinucleated giant cells surrounded by lymphocytes, monocytes and fibroblasts along lymphatic distribution

Staging
- Stage 0 – Normal chest radiograph (5–15%, at presentation)
- Stage 1 – Lymphadenopathy (45-65%)
- Stage 2 – Lymphadenopathy and lung opacities (30-40%)
- Stage 3 – Lung opacities (10-15%)
- Stage 4 – Fibrosis with or without lymphadenopathy (5-25%)

Clinical Issues
Presentation
- Onset – usually age 20 to 40
- Asymptomatic, or fatigue, malaise, weight loss, fever, respiratory symptoms, erythema nodosum, uveitis, skin lesions, arthropathy
- In < 2% TB precedes sarcoidosis or develops later
- Anemia, leukopenia, elevated sed rate, hypercalcemia, nephrolithiasis
- Cutaneous anergy
- Raised ACE level, not specific
- Diagnosis from lung, lymph nodes, and liver biopsy
- Transbronchial biopsy – positive in 90% of cases, even if chest x-ray is normal
- BAL – increased CD4/CD8 ratio, nonspecific finding

Treatment
- Usually not treated; steroids in severe cases
- Recurrence in transplanted lung has been reported

Prognosis
- 80% of cases resolve completely; fibrosis develops in 20%
- Worse in blacks
- Mortality: 2-7%; death respiratory failure, cor pulmonale, hemorrhage

Selected References
1. Traill ZC et al: High-resolution CT findings of pulmonary sarcoidosis. AJR 168:1557-60, 1997
2. Miller BH et al: Thoracic sarcoidosis: Radiologic-pathologic correlation. Radiographics 15:421-37, 1995
3. Rockoff SD et al: Unusual manifestations of thoracic sarcoidosis. AJR 144:513-28, 1985

Langerhans Cell Histiocytosis

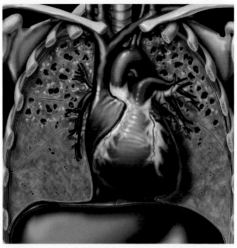

Langerhans cell histiocytosis. Solid nodules, cavitary nodules and thin walled cysts in upper and mid lungs. The cysts may be septated or lobulated and typically have visible thin walls. Sparing of the costophrenic angles is typical of LCH. The differential diagnosis includes LAM.

Key Facts
- Synonyms: Eosinophilic granuloma or histiocytosis X
- Diffuse destructive disorder of distal airways caused by granulomas containing Langerhans cells
- Smoking-related lung disease
- May present with pneumothorax (20%)
- Upper and mid lung reticulonodular opacities, sparing costophrenic angles
- HRCT: Irregular, small nodules and bizarre shaped cysts
- Variable prognosis

Imaging Findings
General Features
- Best imaging clue: Upper lobe nodules and cysts in smoker
Chest Radiograph
- Upper and mid lung reticulonodular opacities, spares costophrenic angles
- Multiple ill-defined nodules, measuring 1-15 mm
- Cysts, honeycombing, blebs, bullae
- Increased lung volumes
- May see rib involvement: Lytic expansile lesion with beveled edges
- No pleural effusion
- 2/3 of patients eventually have resolution or stable disease
CT Findings
- HRCT findings may be characteristic
- Upper and mid lung predominance, spares costophrenic angles
- Irregular centrilobular nodules (usually 1-10 mm), some cavitate
- Cysts (1–20 mm) with thin or thick walls, lobulated, septated, or bizarre shapes
- Ground-glass opacities, interstitial lines, septal lines
- Burned out disease may resemble emphysema

Langerhans Cell Histiocytosis

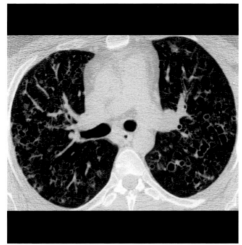

HRCT Langerhans Cell Histiocytosis. Primarily involve the upper lobes. Micronodular centriacinar opacities eventually evolve into thin-walled cysts as demonstrated here. Cysts may coalesce into bizarre shapes. The cysts predispose to spontaneous pneumothorax.

Imaging Recommendations
- HRCT to investigate upper lobe interstitial lung disease, may obviate biopsy in patients with characteristic findings

Differential Diagnosis
Lymphangioleiomyomatosis (LAM)
- LAM has no nodules, round cysts are uniformly distributed, involves costophrenic angles
- Chylothorax
Laryngotracheal Papillomatosis
- Laryngeal and tracheal nodules
- Cysts usually lower lobes and dorsal aspect of lung
Sarcoid
- Often upper lobe, nodules located in lymphatics and will also be seen along pleura, unusual for nodules of Langerhans cell histiocytosis (LCH)
- No cysts
Silicosis
- Often upper lobe, nodules located in lymphatics and will also be seen along pleura
- No cysts
- Egg-shell calcification lymph nodes
Farmer's Lung
- May be upper lobe, also spares costophrenic angles
- Nodules identical to LCH
- No cysts

Langerhans Cell Histiocytosis

Pathology
General
- Diffuse destructive disorder of distal airways caused by granulomas containing Langerhans cells
- Etiology-pathogenesis-pathophysiology
  - Smoking-related lung disease (95% smoke)
  - Langerhans cell processes antigen, contain Birbeck granules
  - LCH probably an allergic reaction to some constituent of smoke
  - Associated with lymphoma, leukemia and solid tumors
  - In adult, LCH most commonly seen only in lung
  - Hand-Schüller-Christian Disease: Involves lung, bone and pituitary – diabetes insipidus (adults and adolescents)
  - Letterer-Siwe: Multiorgan involvement (infants), represents malignant Langerhans cells, poor prognosis

Gross Pathologic-Surgical Features
- End stage fibrosis, honeycombing, cysts and emphysema

Microscopic Features
- 1–15 mm nodules (granulomas) in walls of small airways
- Nodule cavities are due to distended airways
- Adjacent lung may show desquamative interstitial pneumonitis (DIP), bronchiolitis obliterans-organizing pneumonia (BOOP) and respiratory bronchiolitis

Clinical Issues
Presentation
- Uncommon
- White adults, mostly at ages 20–30, heavy smokers, males = females
- Cough, dyspnea, chest pain, fever, weight loss, or asymptomatic (20%)
- May present with pneumothorax (20%) or develop recurrent pneumothoraces
- Diagnosis: Transbronchial lung biopsy, bronchioalveolar lavage (BAL) with $\geq$ 5% CD1A positive Langerhans cells, and or HRCT; open lung biopsy if all else fails

Treatment
- Smoking cessation
- Steroids if disease is progressing

Prognosis
- May recur in transplanted lung
- Variable prognosis from complete remission to respiratory failure
- Mortality is < 5%, worse in men, old age and in patients with recurrent pneumothoraces

Selected References
1. Brauner MW et al: Pulmonary Langerhans cell histiocytosis: Evolution of lesions on CT scans. Radiology 204:497-502, 1997
2. Moore AD et al: Pulmonary histiocytosis X: Comparison of radiographic and CT findings. Radiology 172: 249-54, 1989
3. Friedman PJ et al: Eosinophilic granuloma of lung. Clinical aspects of primary histiocytosis in the adult. Medicine (Baltimore) 60:385-96, 1981

Asbestosis

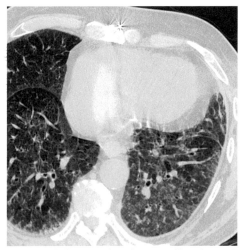

HRCT asbestosis. Multiple short intralobular lines extend from the centriacinar region perpendicularly to the pleural surface. Multiple ground glass opacities and centriacinar nodules. Predominant findings develop in the lower lobes.

Key Facts
- Pneumoconiosis from fibrous silicate minerals
- Peripheral lower zone irregular opacities
- 25% have associated pleural plaques
- HRCT
  - Subpleural curvilinear lines
  - Interlobular lines (short) and parenchymal (long) lines
  - Centriacinar nodules (peribronchial fibrosis)

Imaging Findings
General Features
- Best imaging clue: Basilar honeycombing in patient with pleural plaques
Chest Radiograph
- May be normal
- Peripheral lower zone predominance
- Irregular reticular opacities
- ILO classification: s, t, u opacities
- Late: Endstage honeycombing
- May have pleural plaques (25%)
- Lung cancer: Lower zone predominance
HRCT Findings
- More sensitive than chest radiograph
- Interlobular septal thickening (short lines)
- Subpleural lines
- Parenchymal bands
- Centriacinar nodules (peribronchial fibrosis)
- Honeycombing
- Ground-glass opacities nonspecific
  - Atelectasis (reversible prone position) or early fibrosis

Asbestosis

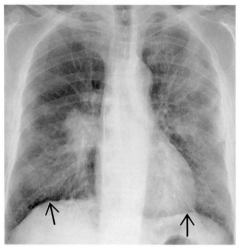

Asbestosis. Multiple Kerley lines lower lobes. Calcified diaphragmatic (arrows) and chest wall plaques. Mass right hilum: Non-small cell carcinoma. The risk of lung cancer in asbestosis equivalent to that of a heavy smoker.

Imaging Recommendations
- HRCT for detection and characterization

Differential Diagnosis
Idiopathic Pulmonary Fibrosis
- No pleural plaques, interstitial thickening identical
Scleroderma
- No plaques, dilated esophagus, interstitial thickening identical
Rheumatoid Arthritis
- No plaques, joint erosions, interstitial thickening identical
Hypersensitivity Pneumonitis
- No plaques, may spare costophrenic angles
Lymphangitic Tumor
- Asymmetric, nodular septal thickening, no plaques
Cytotoxic Drug Reaction
- No plaques, interstitial thickening identical

Pathology
General
- Fibrosis + asbestos bodies = asbestosis
- 2 types of fibers
  - Serpentine (chrysotile, 90% commercial asbestos)
    - Curly, wavy fiber
    - Long (> 100 μm)
    - Diameter (20-40 μm)
  - Amphibole (amosite, crocidolite)
    - Straight, rigid fiber
    - Variable length diameter
    - Aspect ratio (length/width) > 3:1

Asbestosis

- Retention: Long thin fibers > short, thick fibers
- Asbestos (ferruginous) bodies
  o Hemosiderin-coated fiber (mostly amphibole)
  o Incompletely phagocytized by macrophages
  o Not pathognomonic for asbestosis
  o Coated fibers < uncoated fibers
  o Not correlated with fibrosis
- Epidemiology
  o Long - term exposure to asbestos fibers: Mills, insulation, shipyards, construction

Gross Pathologic-Surgical Features
- Coarse honeycombing and volume loss particularly of lower lobes

Microscopic Features
- Early fibrosis: Centered on respiratory bronchioles
- Patchy distribution
- Fibrosis associated with > 1 million fibers/gm lung tissue
  o Honeycombing: Subpleural distribution

Clinical Issues

Presentation
- Gradual onset SOB and dyspnea, nonproductive cough

Natural History
- Latent period 20-30 years
- Multiplicative risk factor for lung cancer
- Clinical diagnosis (4 of 5 criteria)
  o Exposure history
  o Dyspnea on exertion
  o Inspiratory crackles
  o Abnormal compatible chest radiograph
  o Restrictive pattern pulmonary function tests

Treatment
- No treatment, stop smoking, consider lung cancer screening

Prognosis
- High proportion die of lung cancer

Selected References
1. Aberle DR et al: Computed tomography of asbestos-related pulmonary parenchymal and pleural diseases. Clin Chest Med 12:115-31, 1991
2. Akira M et al: Early asbestosis: Evaluation with high-resolution CT. Radiology 178: 409-16, 1991

Progressive Systemic Sclerosis

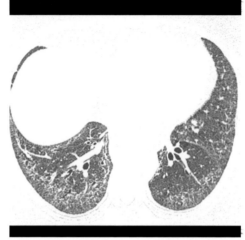

Scleroderma. Non-specific interstitial pneumonia (NSIP) at biopsy. HRCT lung base. Fine "lace-like" interstitial thickening in the subpleural lung. Secondary pulmonary lobule contains numerous intralobular lines and nodules.

Key Facts
- Generalized connective tissue disorder, synonym: Scleroderma
- Symmetric basal reticulonodular pattern ("lace like") with cysts (1 to 30 mm) and/or honeycombing, small volume lungs, air-filled esophagus
- Complications: Renal failure, pulmonary artery hypertension, cardiac disease, lung cancer (alveolar cell and adenocarcinoma), aspiration pneumonia, esophageal disorders, and follicular bronchiolitis, bronchiolitis obliterans organizing pneumonia (BOOP)
- Antinuclear antibodies (100%)
- Prognosis, 70% 5-year survival; cause of death aspiration pneumonia

Imaging Findings
General Features
- Best imaging clue: Basilar interstitial thickening with dilated esophagus
Chest Radiograph
- Abnormal in 20% to 65%
- Progression of fine basilar reticulation ("lace like") to coarse fibrosis
- Widespread symmetric basal reticulonodular pattern with cysts (1 to 30 mm) and/or honeycombing
- Decreased lung volumes, sometimes out of proportion to lung disease
- Elevated diaphragms may also be due to diaphragmatic muscle atrophy and fibrosis
- Dilated, air-filled esophagus without an air-fluid level best seen on lateral
- Pleural thickening and effusions, rare (< 15%)
- Musculoskeletal: Superior and posterolateral rib erosion (< 20%); Absorption distal phalanges, tuft calcification
Esophogram
- Dilated, aperistaltic esophagus
CT/HRCT Findings
- HRCT more sensitive than chest radiography

Progressive Systemic Sclerosis

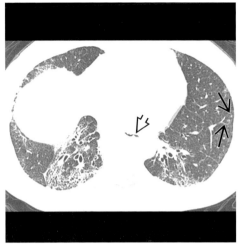

HRCT scleroderma lung base. Fibrosis predominately posterior basilar segments. Traction bronchiectasis subsegmental airways. Ground-glass centriacinar nodules (arrows). Distal esophagus (open arrow) is dilated.

- Peripheral posterior basilar distribution
- Wide spectrum from ground-glass opacities and micronodules to honeycombing
- Lymphadenopathy (60%), esophageal dilatation (80%)
- Pleural thickening (pseudoplaques, 33%)
- Pulmonary artery hypertension, (< 50%) may be separate from interstitial lung disease (ILD)

Imaging Recommendations
- HRCT more sensitive for pulmonary disease; esophogram for motility

Differential Diagnosis

Usual Interstitial Pneumonia (UIP)
- Lacks esophageal dilatation or musculoskeletal changes

Asbestosis
- Pleural plaques, lacks esophageal dilatation, erosion distal clavicles

Rheumatoid Arthritis
- Lacks esophageal dilatation

Drug Reaction
- Lacks esophageal dilatation

Sarcoid
- Lacks esophageal dilatation; Parenchymal findings mid-upper lung

Pathology

General
- Overproduction and tissue deposition of collagen
- Lung fourth most common organ involved after skin, arteries, esophagus
- Etiology-pathogenesis
  - Suspect genetic susceptibility and/or environmental factors
  - Reduced circulating T-suppressor cells and natural killer cells which can suppress fibroblast proliferation

- o Antitopoisomerase I (30%), anti-RNA polymerase III and antihistone antibodies associated with interstitial lung disease
- o Anticentromere antibodies in CREST variant associated with absence of interstitial lung disease
- Epidemiology
  - o Usual onset age 30 to 50; female to male ratio, 3:1; whites=blacks
  - o Uncommon 1.2/100,000

Gross Pathologic-Surgical Features
- Interstitial fibrosis subpleural regions of lower lobes that can progress to end-stage lung (identical to UIP)
- Pleural fibrosis, infrequently identified radiographically

Microscopic Features
- UIP: Fibroblast proliferation, fibrosis and architectural distortion
- NSIP: Cellular or fibrotic
- Follicular bronchiolitis and BOOP
- Vascular changes in small vessels – intimal proliferation, medial hypertrophy, myxomatous changes may lead to pulmonary hypertension

Clinical Issues
Presentation
- Tightening, induration and thickening of the skin, Raynaud's phenomenon, vascular abnormalities, musculoskeletal manifestations, visceral involvement of lungs, heart, and kidneys
- Dyspnea (60%), cough, pleuritic pain, fever, hemoptysis, dysphagia
- Major criteria: Involvement of skin proximal to metacarpophalangeal joints
- Minor criteria: Sclerodactyly, pitting scars, loss of finger tip tufts, bilateral pulmonary basal fibrosis
- Most common presentation is Raynaud's phenomenon (up to 90%), tendonitis, arthralgia, arthritis
- Esophageal dysmotility, gastroesophageal reflux, esophageal candidiasis, and stricture, weight loss
- Antinuclear antibodies (100%)
- PFTs: Restrictive or obstructive defect, decreased diffusion capacity
- BAL varies from lymphocytic to neutrophilic alveolitis (50%)
- Scleroderma features seen in
  - o CREST, MCTD, diffuse fasciitis and eosinophilia, carcinoid syndrome, drug reactions, chronic graft versus host disease

Natural History
- Lung disease indolent and progressive
- Complications: Renal failure, pulmonary artery hypertension and cardiac disease, lung cancer, (alveolar cell and adenocarcinoma), and aspiration pneumonia

Treatment & Prognosis
- No specific treatment
- Renal failure may actually improve musculoskeletal disease
- Poor; 70% 5-year survival; cause of death usually aspiration pneumonia

Selected References
1. Bhalla M et al: Chest CT in patients with scleroderma: Prevalence of asymptomatic esophageal dilatation. AJR 161: 269-72, 1993
2. Schurawitzki H et al: Interstitial lung disease in progressive systemic sclerosis: High-resolution CT versus radiography. Radiology 176:755-9, 1990

Rheumatoid Arthritis

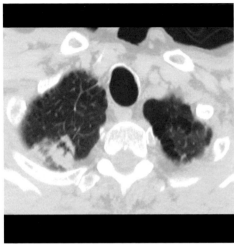

Rheumatoid nodule. Subpleural partially cavitated nodule right apex. Paraseptal emphysema. Rheumatoid nodules may produce a pneumothorax.

Key Facts
- Subacute or chronic inflammatory polyarthropathy of unknown cause
- Thoracic involvement more common in males
- Major findings are pleural disease, interstitial fibrosis with honeycombing, micronodules, small and large nodules, and airway disease
- HRCT useful to investigate pleuropulmonary and airway disease
- Interstitial lung disease: Usual Interstitial Pneumonia (UIP) or non-specific interstial pneumonia (NSIP), the latter having a better prognosis
- Treatment - steroids and immunosuppressive drugs
- Complications include pneumonia, empyema, drug reaction, amyloid, cor pulmonale

Imaging Findings
General Features
- Best imaging clue: Diffuse interstitial thickening with erosion distal clavicles

Chest Radiograph
- Pleural Disease
  - Pleural thickening (20%)
  - Pleural effusion, mostly in males (3%)
    - Small to large, usually unilateral, can be bilateral
    - Transient, persistent or relapsing
    - Fibrothorax
    - Susceptible to empyema
  - Pneumothorax – rare
- Parenchymal Disease
  - Reticulonodular and irregular linear opacities, lower zones (< 10%)
  - Distortion, honeycombing, progressive loss of volume
  - Upper lobe fibrobullous disease, rare
  - Rheumatoid nodules, rare
    - Solitary or multiple, 5 mm to 7 cm

Rheumatoid Arthritis

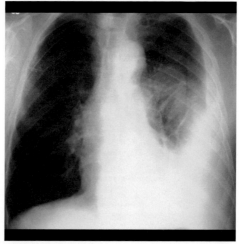

Rheumatoid pleural effusion. Moderate sized left pleural effusion. Previous gunshot injury right hemithorax. The pleural effusion was drained but re-accumulated to the same level as before. Pleural fluid both low in glucose and positive for rheumatoid factor.

- Peripheral
- Wax and wane
- May cavitate, thick smooth wall
- May calcify
  - Caplan's syndrome – rare
    - Hypersensitivity reaction to dust
    - Coal miners, large rounded nodules (0.5 to 5 cm)
    - Redefined to include: Silica, asbestos, dolomite, carbon
    - Serologic and not clinical RA
- Airway Disease
  - Hyperinflation (bronchiolitis obliterans) or BOOP pattern
  - Diffuse reticulonodular pattern - Follicular bronchiolitis
  - Bronchiectasis

HRCT Findings
- Pleural disease - most common
  - Pleural thickening or effusion
  - May be associated with pericarditis, interstitial fibrosis, interstitial pneumonia or lung nodules
- Parenchymal disease
  - Pulmonary fibrosis indistinguishable from UIP
    - Honeycombing (10%), mostly at bases
    - Ground-glass opacities (15%)
  - Consolidation (5%)
  - Micronodules (20%) (centrilobular, peribronchial, subpleural)
  - Nodules/masses
    - Resemble neoplasm, discrete, rounded or lobulated, subpleural
- Airway disease
  - Mosaic perfusion, BOOP pattern, bronchiectasis

Rheumatoid Arthritis

- o Micronodules < 1 cm; centrilobular, subpleural, peribronchial; centrilobular branching pattern in follicular bronchiolitis
- Other findings
  - o Cor pulmonale, lymphadenopathy, sclerosing mediastinitis, pericarditis

<u>Imaging Recommendations</u>
- HRCT useful to characterize pattern and extent of disease

Differential Diagnosis
<u>General</u>
- Hand films or chest radiographic findings in distal clavicles (erosions) useful to differentiate RA from other interstitial lung diseases

<u>Lung</u>
- Idiopathic pulmonary fibrosis (IPF), scleroderma, asbestosis, drug reaction, hypersensitivity pneumonitis may have identical pulmonary findings

Pathology
<u>General</u>
- Subacute or chronic inflammatory polyarthropathy of unknown cause
- Etiology-pathogenesis
  - o Possible inflammatory, immunologic, hormonal, and genetic factors
- Epidemiolgy: RA is 3x more common in females

<u>Microscopic Features</u>
- Pulmonary fibrosis, either UIP or NSIP pattern
- Pleural biopsy – may show rheumatoid nodules
- Pleural fluid - lymphocytes, acutely neutrophils and eosinophils

Clinical Issues
<u>Presentation</u>
- Extraarticular RA - more common in males, age 50-60 years
- Thoracic disease may develop before, at onset or after onset of arthritis
- Insidious onset, with relapses and remissions
- Asymptomatic, or dyspnea, cough, pleuritic pain, finger clubbing, hemoptysis, infection, bronchopleural fistula, pneumothorax
- Most have arthritis; positive rheumatoid factor (80%), and cutaneous nodules
- Pleural fluid - high protein, low glucose, low pH, high LDH, high RF, low complement
- PFTs - restrictive defect, reduced diffusing capacity, sometimes obstructive defect if predominant airways disease

<u>Treatment</u>
- Treatment: Steroids, immunosuppressant drugs

<u>Prognosis</u>
- 5-year survival 40%
- Death from infection, respiratory failure, cor pulmonale, amyloidosis

Selected References
1. Remy-Jardin M et al: Lung changes in rheumatoid arthritis: CT findings. Radiology 193: 375-82, 1994
2. Turner-Warwick M et al: Pulmonary manifestations of rheumatoid disease. Clin Rheum Dis 3:549-64, 1977

Sjogren's Syndrome

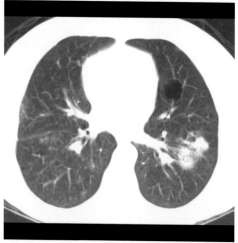

HRCT Sjogren's syndrome. Peribronchovascular nodules and larger airspace mass left lower lobe. Thin walled cystic lesion in lingula. Biopsy proven lymphocytic interstitial pneumonia.

Key Facts
- Autoimmune disorder primarily affects middle-aged females
- Commonly associated with other connective tissue diseases (secondary Sjogren's syndrome (SS)
- Widespread tissue infiltration by polyclonal B-lymphocytes
- Keratoconjunctivitis sicca, xerostomia, recurrent swelling of the parotid gland
- Radiography: Interstitial lung disease (UIP, LIP), cystic lung disease, recurrent pneumonias, airway disease
- Increased risk for pseudolymphoma and lymphoma

Imaging Findings
General Features
- Best imaging clue: Thin-walled cysts rare
Chest Radiograph
- Chest radiograph abnormal in < 33%
- Reticulonodular pattern, basal predominance (most common)
- Bronchial wall thickening, bronchiectasis
- Recurrent bronchopneumonias
- Atelectasis
- Pleural effusion or thickening (uncommon)
- Pulmonary artery hypertension (uncommon)
- Lymphadenopathy suggests pseudolymphoma or malignant lymphoma
HRCT Findings
- Basal predominance
- Bronchiolectasis, centrilobular nodules or branching opacities
- Mosaic attenuation, air trapping
- Thin-walled cysts (5-30 mm)
- Linear opacities (septal and nonseptal)
- Airspace opacities – bronchopneumonia or pseudolymphoma

Sjogren's Syndrome

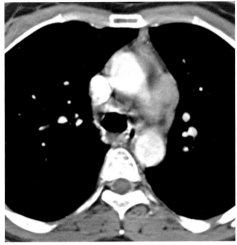

Sjogren's syndrome. New mediastinal adenopathy in the aortico-pulmonary window. Non-Hodgkins lymphoma, patients with Sjogren's are a risk for developing this neoplasm.

- Pleural effusion or thickening (uncommon)

Differential Diagnosis

Usual Interstitial Pneumonia (UIP)
- Lacks thin-walled cysts, subpleural interstitial thickening

Drug Reaction
- Lacks thin-walled cysts

Asbestosis
- Pleural plaques, lacks thin-walled cysts, long and short parenchymal lines

Langerhans Cell Granulomatosis
- Cysts predominately upper lobes, small centriacinar nodules

Lymphangiomyomatosis
- Cysts more diffuse, pleural effusion, spontaneous pneumothorax

Pneumocystis Carinii Pneumonia
- Cysts (pneumatoceles) follow PCP infection

Pathology

General
- Autoimmune process
- Etiology-pathogenesis
  - Possible viral etiology: EB, hepatitis C, herpes 6, retrovirus

Gross Pathologic-Surgical Features
- Lymphocytic infiltration, glandular atrophy, impaired secretion of lacrimal, salivary, airway mucous glands
- Pleuropulmonary abnormalities (30%)
  - Airway disease
    - Tracheobronchitis
    - Follicular bronchiolitis
    - BOOP

- o Recurrent pneumonias
- o Interstitial lung disease (33%)
  - Lymphocytic interstitial pneumonia (LIP) (diffuse)
  - Pseudolymphoma (localized)
  - UIP pattern
- o Pleuritis with or without effusion, pleural thickening (10%)
- o Lymphadenitis
- o Plexogenic pulmonary arteriopathy (rare)
- o Amyloidosis as a secondary manifestation

<u>Microscopic Features</u>
- Infiltration of tissues with polyclonal B-lymphocytes
- Systemic necrotizing vasculitis, small and large vessels

Clinical Issues
<u>Presentation</u>
- Females (90%), mean age 57 years
- Sicca syndrome: Dry eyes, mouth, nose
- Hoarseness, cough, pleuritic pain, dyspnea
- Lacrimal, submandibular and parotid gland enlargement
- Recurrent infections, bronchitis, pneumonia (secondary to impaired secretions)
- Associated with other autoimmune diseases: Chronic active hepatitis, primary biliary cirrhosis, Hashimoto's thyroiditis, myasthenia gravis, celiac disease, renal tubular disorders, myopathy, neuropathy, CNS disorders, Raynaud's, vasculitis, purpura, polyarthropathy, thrombocytopenic purpura (rare), hypothyroidism, splenomegaly
- Secondary SS associated with rheumatoid arthritis, progressive systemic sclerosis (PSS), systemic lupus erythematosus (SLE), polymyositis
- Positive rheumatoid factor (90%), ANA (70%)
- Lymphopenia, leukopenia, polyclonal gammopathy IgG, IgM
- Diagnosis
  - o Sicca syndrome
  - o Abnormal Schirmer's test/Rose Bengal test
  - o Biopsy of minor salivary glands
  - o Parotid sialography
  - o Detection of antibodies to extractable nuclear antigens (SS-A, SS-B)
- PFTs – obstructive (maybe reversible) or restrictive, decreased diffusion
- Bronchioalveolar lavage (BAL) – lymphocytosis

<u>Treatment</u>
- None, supportive
- Radiation and chemotherapy for lymphoma

<u>Prognosis</u>
- Primary SS, may progress rapidly with poor prognosis
- Risk for non-Hodgkin's lymphoma or pseudolymphoma

Selected References
1.   Meyer CA et al: Inspiratory and expiratory high-resolution CT findings in a patient with Sjogren's syndrome and cystic lung disease. AJR 168:101-3, 1997
2.   Strimlan CV et al: Pulmonary manifestations of Sjogren's syndrome. Chest 70:354-61, 1976

Hypersensitivity Pneumonitis

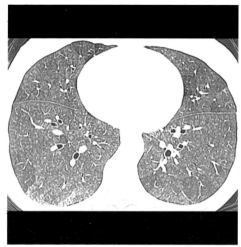

Farmer's lung. HRCT through midlung. Patchy, centrilobular, ground-glass opacities, and micronodules.

Key Facts
- Chest usually normal in acute, subacute disease
- Midlung fibrosis in chronic disease
- HRCT: Centrilobular ground-glass nodules with air trapping
- Usually spares costophrenic angles
- Allergic reaction to organic antigens especially thermophilic actinomycetes
- Nonspecific flu-like symptoms
- Often misdiagnosed as "pneumonia"

Imaging Findings
General Features
- Best imaging clue: Midlung miliary or interstitial disease, sparing costophrenic angles

Chest Radiograph
- Often normal, especially acute and subacute forms
- Miliary disease
- Chronic: Midlung to upper lung zone fibrosis, bronchiectasis, and volume loss
- No pleural disease or adenopathy

HRCT Findings
- More sensitive but may be normal
- Ground-glass centrilobular nodules acutely
- Most prominent mid to lower lungs
- Air trapping common (mosaic perfusion pattern)
- Spares costophrenic angles

Imaging Recommendations
- HRCT more sensitive and best to characterize disease

Differential Diagnosis
Idiopathic Pulmonary Fibrosis
- Does not spare costophrenic angles, in fact, usually severely involved

107

Hypersensitivity Pneumonitis

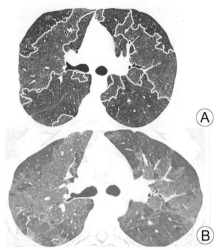

Farmer's lung. HRCT midlung at inspiration and expiration. Inspiration (A) mosaic perfusion (white outline). Hypoattenuation predominately peripheral. Expiration (B) mixed attenuation, combination of both small airways obstruction and ground glass infiltration.

<u>Eosinophilic Granuloma</u>
- Nodules may cavitate, not seen with HP
- Smokers (HP rare in smokers)

<u>Sarcoid</u>
- Peribronchovascular distribution, subpleural nodules, adenopathy

<u>Pneumoconiosis</u>
- Occupational history
- May have adenopathy
- Subpleural lymphatic deposits rare in hypersensitivity pneumonitis (HP)

<u>Scleroderma</u>
- Dilated esophagus, basilar fibrosis

Pathology

<u>General</u>
- Allergic reaction to airborne organic particles (1-5 um)
- Etiology-Pathogenesis
  - Thermophilic actinomycetes common antigen
  - Small particles deposit in bronchioles, incite allergic granulomatous reaction

<u>Gross Pathologic-Surgical Features</u>
- Honeycomb lung in chronic HP
- Distribution mid to upper lung
- Costophrenic angles less involved

<u>Microscopic Features</u>
- Loosely-formed, noncaseating granulomas
- Lymphocytic infiltration
- BOOP

Hypersensitivity Pneumonitis

Clinical Issues

Presentation
- Typical exposure
  - Wet hay: Farmer's lung
  - Birds: Pigeon-breeder's lung
  - Office: Humidifier lung
  - Numerous other organic antigens identified (i.e. mushrooms, etc.)
- Acute, subacute, chronic forms, considerable overlap
- Nonspecific symptoms
- Often mistaken as pneumonia
- Acute: Cough, dyspnea, fever 4-6 hours following exposure
- Subacute or chronic: Insidious onset of SOB or dyspnea
- Individual must be susceptible (allergic response), most dust-exposed individuals have no response

Treatment
- Removal from environment
- Steroids

Prognosis
- Variable, complete recovery with removal of antigen to endstage fibrosis

Selected References
1. Matar LD et al: Hypersensitivity pneumonitis. AJR 174:1061-6, 2000
2. Lynch DA et al: Can CT distinguish hypersensitivity pneumonitis from idiopathic pulmonary fibrosis? AJR 165:807-11, 1995

Pneumoconiosis, Coal and Silica

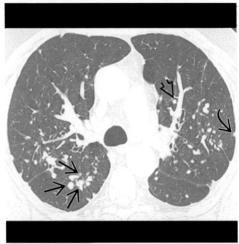

Silicosis. HRCT midlung. Multiple nodules predominately in the dorsal aspect of the lung. Nodules located along bronchovascular bundles (open arrow) and subpleural lungs (curved arrow). Aggregation of nodules may represent early PMF (arrows).

Key Facts
- Miners inhaling quartz (silica) or coal dust
- Simple pneumoconiosis: Micronodules < 1 cm, upper lungs, hilar/ mediastinal lymphadenopathy, eggshell calcifications
- Complicated pneumoconiosis known as progressive massive fibrosis (PMF): Aggregation of nodules into large masses, may cavitate
- As PMF worsens, profusion of nodules decreases
- Acute silicoproteinosis: Resembles alveolar proteinosis
- Caplan's syndrome: Coal worker's pneumoconiosis (CWP) + rheumatoid arthritis + necrobiotic nodules

Imaging Findings
General Features
- Best imaging clue: Micronodular interstitial thickening in upper lung zones
Chest Radiograph
- Findings seen 10 to 20 years after exposure
- Silicosis and CWP similar, lung disease usually less severe in CWP
- Simple pneumoconiosis
  - 1–3 mm nodules, posterior segments, upper lobes (ILO p,q,r)
  - Nodules may calcify
  - Hilar and mediastinal lymphadenopathy, eggshell calcification
- Complicated pneumoconiosis (PMF)
  - Nodules coalesce and are > 1 cm in diameter
  - Usually bilateral, right > left, in dorsal aspect of lung
  - PMF may be lens shaped (wide PA and narrow lateral view)
  - Overall profusion of nodules decreases due to aggregation into PMF
  - May have foci of amorphous calcification, may cavitate
  - Migrates centrally with time
  - Lung distal to PMF emphysematous: Risk for pneumothorax
- Acute silicoproteinosis

Pneumoconiosis, Coal and Silica

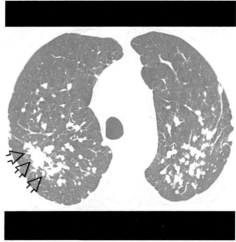

Complicated silicosis. HRCT upper lobes. Multiple nodules aggregating into PMF in the dorsal aspect of right upper lobe (open arrows). Multiple subpleural nodules.

- o Butterfly alveolar proteinosis pattern with air bronchograms
- o Hilar/mediastinal lymphadenopathy
- o Progresses rapidly over months
- o Later fibrosis, distortion, bullae, pneumothorax
- Caplan's syndrome
  - o Multiple large nodules (may cavitate)
  - o Nodular interstitial thickening (CWP)
  - o Bone changes of rheumatoid arthritis: Humeral or clavicular erosions

HRCT Findings
- More sensitive than chest radiography
- Micronodules < 7 mm in center and periphery of lobule, may calcify
- Aggregation of nodules into PMF more readily detected

Imaging Recommendations
- HRCT more sensitive for pulmonary disease and PMF

Differential Diagnosis
Sarcoidosis
- No occupational exposure, PMF less likely

Tuberculosis (TB)
- Nodules do not aggregate into mass, profusion nodules less

Langerhans Cell Histiocytosis
- Less likely subpleural nodules, no PMF, cysts

Hypersensitivity Pneumonitis
- Less likely subpleural nodules, no PMF, primarily midlung

Pathology
General
- Increased risk of tuberculosis
- Silica more fibrogenic than coal
- Etiology-pathogenesis

Pneumoconiosis, Coal and Silica

  o Inhalation of silica dust, silicon dioxide (SiO_2) or coal, deposited in respiratory bronchioles, removed by macrophages and lymphatics

Gross Pathologic-Surgical Features
- Primarily involves upper lung zones, PMF results in end-stage lung

Microscopic Features
- Silica particles within concentric lamellae of collagen in bronchioles, small vessels, and lymphatics
- Birefringent silicate crystals (1–3 µ) in nodules by polarized microscopy
- Silica-laden macrophages carry particles to hilar and mediastinal nodes and form granulomas
- Silicoproteinosis high concentrations of silica, alveolar filling by lipoproteinaceous material, similar to alveolar proteinosis
- Coal macule: Stellate collection of macrophages containing black particles, (1-5 µ) in terminal and respiratory bronchioles and pleural lymphatics

Clinical Issues
Presentation
- Occupations: Sandblasting, quarries, mining, glassblowing, pottery
- Coal mines usually contain silica (most common element, earth's crust)
- Acute silicoproteinosis
  o Massive exposure to silica dust, usually seen in sandblasters
- Caplan's syndrome
  o CWP, rheumatoid arthritis, necrobiotic lung nodules
- Symptoms
  o None with simple silicosis
  o Miners commonly smoke and have bronchitis or emphysema
  o Cough, dyspnea, increased sputum in complicated disease
  o Black sputum in coal workers
- PFTs – decreased diffusion capacity, obstructive, then restrictive defect
- At risk for tuberculosis; cavitation in PMF requires culture
- Slight increased risk of lung cancer, scleroderma

Natural History
- Usually requires > 20 years exposure, silicosis progressive even after removal of dust, CWP usually not progressive

Treatment
- Removal from work environment
- Prevention, respirators in dusty environment, dust control

Prognosis
- Simple, normal longevity
- Complicated PMF, death from respiratory failure, pneumothorax, carcinoma, TB
- Silicoproteinosis: Death within 2 to 3 years

Selected References
1. Remy-Jardin M et al: Coal worker's pneumoconiosis: CT assessment in exposed workers and correlation with radiographic findings. Radiology 177:363-71, 1990
2. Bergin CJ et al: CT in silicosis: Correlation with plain films and pulmonary function tests. AJR 146:477-83, 1986
3. Pendergrass EP: Some considerations concerning the roentgen diagnosis of pneumoconiosis and silicosis. AJR 48:571-94, 1942

Ankylosing Spondylitis

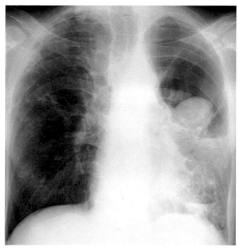

Ankylosing spondylitis, Extensive fibrobullous disease in both upper lobes. Left upper lobe bulla contains an aspergilloma. Aorta normal.

Key Facts
- Synovitis, sacroiliitis, thoracolumbar spondyloarthritis, ankylosis, kyphosis
- Genetic predisposition: HLA-B27, mostly males, onset 15-35 years
- Pleuropulmonary disease, late onset, rare, usually asymptomatic
- Radiography: Upper lobe fibrobullous disease, cysts, cavities, cicatricial atelectasis, and mycetomas
- Hemoptysis from mycetoma may be life threatening
- Usually, normal life span
- Dilatation ascending aorta and aortic insufficiency

Imaging Findings
General Features
- Best imaging clue: Upper lobe fibrobullous disease with spinal ankylosis
Chest Radiograph
- Upper lobe symmetric fibrobullous disease, rare (1.25%)
- Cicatricial atelectasis and traction bronchiectasis upper lobes
- Stable or slowly progressive
- Cysts and cavities, thick or thin-walled
- Pleural thickening, pneumothorax, 8%
- Superimposed aspergillomas
- Pleural effusion or thickening, rare
- Bone changes
  - Ankylosis nearly always precedes lung disease
  - Kyphosis
  - Syndesmophytes
  - Squared vertebra
  - Eroded or fused manubriosternal joint
  - Ossification of costotransverse joints
- Dilatation ascending aorta and aortic insufficiency
HRCT Findings
- Apical fibrobullous disease

Ankylosing Spondylitis

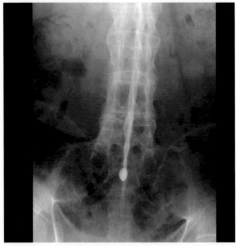

Ankylosing spondylitis. Ankylosis of both sacroiliac joints and lumbar spine. Patient has long history of spinal disease prior to developing lung disease.

- Non-apical interstitial lung disease
  - Ground-glass opacities
  - Basal subpleural bands
  - Thickened interlobular septa
  - Pleural tags
- Bronchial wall thickening, bronchiectasis, tracheal dilatation
- Paraseptal emphysema, cysts, cavities
- Mycetoma
- Lymphadenopathy, mild
- Pleuritis with effusion

Imaging Recommendations
- Chest radiograph sufficient for diagnosis

Differential Diagnosis

Tuberculosis
- Lacks spinal ankylosis
- Requires culture

Histoplasmosis
- Lacks spinal ankylosis
- Requires culture

Sarcoidosis
- Lacks spinal ankylosis

Silicosis and Coal Worker's Pneumoconiosis
- Lacks spinal ankylosis
- Eggshell calcification in hilar and mediastinal lymph nodes
- Occupational history

Pathology

General
- Cavities colonized with fungus balls (Aspergillus fumigatus) or non-tuberculous mycobacterial infection

Ankylosing Spondylitis

- Genetics
  - o Genetic predisposition: HLA-B27

Gross Pathologic-Surgical Features
- Bronchiectasis, tracheobronchomegaly, BOOP
- Bullae

Microscopic Features
- Nonspecific fibrosis, chronic lymphocytic infiltration, elastic fragmentation, collagen degeneration

Clinical Issues

Presentation
- In approximately 1 in 2000; males: female = 8:1
- Intermittent low back pain, chest pain, fatigue, weight loss, low grade fever
- Hemoptysis may be due to mycetomas and may be life-threatening
- Chest wall restriction, kyphosis
- Aortic valvulitis, 5%
- Pleuropulmonary disease, 1-2%
  - o Late onset, 15 to 20 years after spinal disease
  - o Upper lobe fibrobullous disease, asymptomatic
- PFTs: Mixed - hyperinflation or restriction

Treatment
- Aortic valve replacement for valvulitis
- Bronchial artery embolization or surgery for life threatening hemoptysis
- Treat superimposed infection

Prognosis
- Mortality associated with spondylitis, ulcerative colitis, nephritis, TB, respiratory disease
- Usually, normal life span

Selected References
1.   Fenlon HM et al: Plain radiographs and thoracic high-resolution CT in patients with ankylosing spondylitis. AJR 168: 1067-72, 1997
2.   Rosenow E et al: Pleuropulmonary manifestations of ankylosing spondylitis. Mayo Clin Proc 52:641-9, 1977
3.   Wolson AH et al: Upper lobe fibrosis in ankylosing spondylitis. AJR 124:466-71, 1975

Drug Reaction

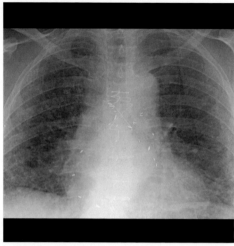

Cardiomegaly and diffuse interstitial thickening. Previous median sternotomy. While edema would be the most likely diagnosis, the interstitial thickening had been chronic and did not respond to diuretics.

Key Facts
- Drug toxicity often overlooked as cause of pulmonary disease
- CT/HRCT can be helpful for toxicity from certain drugs, e.g., amiodarone, steroids, methysergide, mineral oil, vitamin D, talc
- Presentation: Varied, dyspnea, cough, fever, eosinophilia
- Mortality from respiratory failure

Imaging Findings
General Features
- Best imaging clue: High index of suspicion that pulmonary findings may be drug related
Chest Radiograph
- Nonspecific
- Patterns
  o Diffuse interstitial thickening (acute or chronic)
  o Fleeting peripheral consolidation ("eosinophilic pneumonia-like")
  o Granulomas
  o Cavitation (vasculitis)
  o Fine calcification
  o Pleural and pericardial effusions/fibrosis
  o Hilar/mediastinal lymphadenopathy
  o Pneumothorax (cocaine, nitrosoureas)
  o Pneumomediastinum (cocaine)
  o Pulmonary artery hypertension (talc, fenfluramine)
CT/HRCT Findings
- HRCT more sensitive and more specific
- High density CT deposits in lung and liver
  o Amiodarone – contains 37% iodine by weight
- Lipoid pneumonia: Mineral oil ingestion
- Mediastinal lipomatosis/extrapleural fat from steroids

Drug Reaction

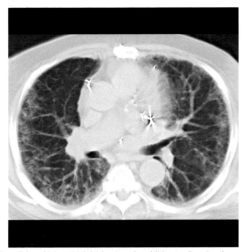

Nonspecific peripheral interstitial thickening. In addition to chronic edema, differential would include UIP, collagen vascular disease, and drug reaction. History of amiodarone therapy. The liver may be dense from amiodarone accumulation (amiodarone contains iodine).

- Metastatic pulmonary calcification from vitamin D

<u>Imaging Recommendations</u>
- CT may be useful for detection (sensitivity) and characterizing opacities

Differential Diagnosis
<u>General</u>
- Nearly any focal or diffuse pulmonary process could potentially be secondary to drug use. Differentiation requires investigation of drug history and an individual's drug's pattern of pulmonary injury

Pathology
<u>General</u>
- Pathogenesis complex
  - Hypersensitivity, acute and chronic
  - Diffuse alveolar damage (DAD) pattern
  - UIP pattern

<u>Microscopic Features</u>
- No specific microscopic features, pattern varies from granulomas to DAD

Clinical Issues
<u>Presentation</u>
- Approximately 40 commonly used drugs may cause lung disease
- Onset: variable from immediate to years after drug initiation
- Symptoms usually nonspecific fever, cough, dyspnea
  - Asthma: Mitomycin
- May have eosinophilia
- Specific drugs
  - Pulmonary edema

Drug Reaction

- ▪ Heroin, cocaine, aspirin, contrast media, cytosine arabinoside, Interleukin-2, hydrochlorothiazide, tricyclic antidepressants
- o Hemolytic uremic syndrome: Mitomycin
- o Diffuse alveolar damage (DAD)
  - ▪ Cytoxan, bleomycin, methotrexate, busulfan, carmustine, oxygen
  - ▪ Bleomycin: Multiple nodules may simulate metastases
- o Pleura/mediastinal fibrosis
  - ▪ Methysergide, ergotamine, ergonovine
- o Pleural effusions
  - ▪ Methotrexate, procarbazine, nitrofurantoin
- o Hypersensitivity reaction (Type I or III)
  - ▪ Bleomycin, methotrexate, procarbazine
- o Neural or humoral mechanisms
  - ▪ Asthma – propranolol, neostigmine, aspirin
- o Autoimmune response, systemic lupus erythematosus, drug-induced
  - ▪ Procainamide, hydralazine, isoniazid, phenytoin
- o Vasculitis
  - ▪ Sulfonamides, penicillin, cromolyn sodium
- o Pulmonary hemorrhage
  - ▪ Anticoagulants, estrogens, penicillamine, and others
- o Drug-induced phospholipidosis: Amiodarone
- o Constrictive bronchiolitis
  - ▪ Penicillamine, sulfasalazine
- o Pulmonary calcification: Vitamin D
- o Chronic pleural effusions/fibrosis: Bromocriptine
- o Hilar/mediastinal lymphadenopathy
  - ▪ Methotrexate, phenytoin
- o Granulomas
  - ▪ Methotrexate, nitrofurantoin, mineral oils, talc

Treatment
- Withdraw drug
- Steroids for DAD

Prognosis
- Recovery after discontinuance of drug
- Potentially fatal
  - o Nitrofurantoin 10% mortality
- Malignant transformation: Dilantin adenopathy may evolve into lymphoma

Selected References
1. Rosenow III EC et al: Drug-induced pulmonary disease. An update. Chest 102:239-50, 1992
2. Rossi SE et al: Pulmonary drug toxicity: Radiologic and pathologic manifestations. Radiographs 20:1245-59, 2000

Lymphangitic Carcinomatosis

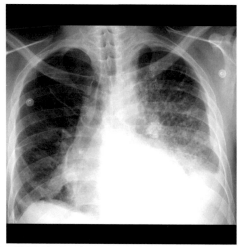

Diffuse interstitial thickening throughout the left lung with relative sparing of the right lung. Moderate to large left pleural effusion and possible cardiomegaly. History of previous lung cancer. Lymphangitic carcinomatosis left lung.

Key Facts
- Permeation of lymphatics by neoplastic cells
- Tumor emboli or direct spread to lungs from hilar nodes or lung cancer mass
- Seen with carcinoma of the lung, breast, pancreas, stomach, colon, prostate and other tumors
- Unilateral disease - most commonly due to lung cancer
- Radiography - may resemble interstitial edema
- HRCT: Nodular thickening of interlobular septa and bronchovascular bundles
- Lung architecture preserved
- Prognosis: Poor

Imaging Findings
General Features
- Best imaging clue: Nodular septal thickening which may spare whole lobes or lung
Chest Radiograph
- Reticulonodular opacities, coarse bronchovascular markings, septal lines, subpleural edema at fissures
- May resemble interstitial edema
- Hilar and mediastinal lymphadenopathy may be present
- Pleural effusion common
- Unilateral disease - most commonly due to lung cancer
- Bilateral symmetric disease commonly due to extrathoracic primary tumor
- Chest radiograph may be normal
CT Findings
- HRCT best imaging to suggest diagnosis
- Nodular thickening of interlobular septa and bronchovascular bundles
- Septal lines and polygons with nodular or beaded appearance

Lymphangitic Carcinomatosis

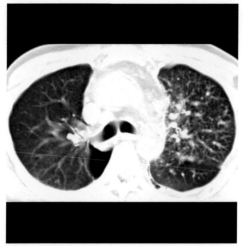

Marked thickening of the bronchovascular bundles in the left lung. Paraseptal emphysema superior segment right lower lobe. Lymphangitic tumor more likely to involve the bronchovascular bundles and spare lobes or lungs. Beaded peripheral septal thickening is also characteristic although it is less common.

- Lung architecture preserved
- Patchy ground-glass and airspace opacities
- Small, centrilobular nodules, thickened centrilobular bronchovascular bundles
- Peripheral or central distribution within lobule, basal predominance
- Commonly asymmetric, may spare lobes or lungs
- Smooth or nodular thickening of interlobar fissures
- Pleural effusion
- Hilar/mediastinal lymphadenopathy

Imaging Recommendations
- HRCT diagnostic features, beaded septal thickening in patient with known malignancy

Differential Diagnosis
General
- Lymphangitic carcinomatosis will not show architectural distortion or honeycombing, progressive disease, usually not occult but develops in patients with known malignancy
- Pleural effusion not seen in sarcoid, HP, asbestosis, or idiopathic interstitial lung disease
Pulmonary Edema
- Rapidly resolves with treatment, cardiomegaly, vascular redistribution
UIP
- Reticular rather than nodular
Scleroderma
- Dilated esophagus, reticular rather than beaded thickening
Drug Reaction
- Drug history, septal thickening usually not nodular or beaded

Lymphangitic Carcinomatosis

Sarcoid
• Adenopathy, peribronchial, septa not usually beaded
Asbestosis
• Pleural plaques, reticular not nodular
Hypersensitivity Pneumonitis
• Antigen exposure, septa not beaded

Pathology
General
• Frequent form of tumor spread
• Permeation of lymphatics by neoplastic cells
• Etiology-pathogenesis
  o 2 pulmonary lymphatic systems: Axial and peripheral
  o Frequency of involvement: Axial > Axial + peripheral > Peripheral
  o Hematogenous metastases: Tumor emboli to small pulmonary artery branches with subsequent spread along lymphatics
  o Some tumors such as lymphoma spread from hilar nodes retrograde into pulmonary lymphatics
  o Lung cancer can spread to adjacent lung along lymphatics
Gross Pathologic-Surgical Features
• Interstitial thickening of interlobular septa due to tumor cells, desmoplastic response, and dilated lymphatics
• Hilar and mediastinal lymph nodes may or may not be involved
Microscopic Features
• Nests of tumor cells within lymphatics, may be associated with fibrosis

Clinical Issues
Presentation
• Seen with carcinoma of the lung, breast, pancreas, stomach, colon, prostate and other tumors
• Dyspnea, cough, progressive symptoms
• Usually not presenting manifestation, usually develops in patients with known malignancy
• If no known malignancy – sputum cytology, transbronchial biopsy, fine needle aspiration biopsy or open lung biopsy for diagnosis
Treatment
• Aimed at underlying malignancy
Prognosis
• Poor, 15% survive 6 months

Selected References
1.   Ren H et al: Computed tomography of inflation-fixed lungs: The beaded septum sign of pulmonary metastases. J Comput Assist Tomogr 13:411-6, 1989
2.   Trapnell DH: Radiological appearance of lymphangitis carcinomatosa of the lung. Thorax 19: 251-60,1964

Systemic Lupus Erythematosus

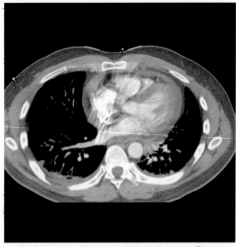

Systemic Lupus Erythematosus (SLE). Small bilateral pleural effusions and pericardial effusion. Serosal inflammation and effusions are the commonest manifestation of lupus.

Key Facts
- Chronic collagen vascular disease primarily in women
- Thoracic manifestations in 70%
- Pleural thickening or effusion most common
- Elevated diaphragms due to diaphragm weakness
- Thromboembolic disease due to antiphospholipid antibodies
- Multiple drugs may result in lupus erythematosus

Imaging Findings
General Features
- Best imaging clue: Unexplained, small, bilateral, pleural effusions or pleural thickening in young women

Chest Radiograph
- Pleural effusion or pleural thickening 50%
  - Usually small, either unilateral or bilateral
- Interstitial pneumonitis resembling UIP
- Elevated diaphragm (diaphragmatic dysfunction) 20%
  - Basilar atelectasis
- Consolidation
  - Pneumonia
  - Hemorrhage
  - Acute lupus pneumonitis
  - Infarcts from thromboembolism
  - Bronchiolitis obliterans organizing pneumonia (BOOP)
- Cardiac enlargement
  - Pericardial effusion
  - Renal failure
- Pulmonary artery hypertension

CT Findings
- More sensitive than chest radiography

Systemic Lupus Erythematosus

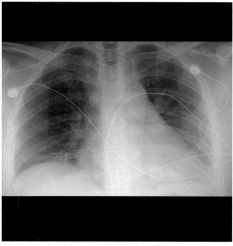

SLE. Lung volumes are low. Heart is mildly enlarged. Decreased lung volumes may be due to diaphragmatic dysfunction. Small pericardial effusion at echocardiography.

- ○ Centriacinar nodules 20%
- ○ Bronchial wall thickening or bronchiectasis 33%
- ○ Mild adenopathy < 2 cm 20%

Differential Diagnosis

Cardiogenic Pulmonary Edema
- • Interstitial thickening less common with SLE

Pneumonia
- • Identical radiographic findings, often seen with SLE

Goodpasture's Syndrome
- • Parenchymal changes more severe than SLE

Usual Interstitial Pneumonia (UIP)
- • Honeycombing, rare with SLE

Nonspecific Interstitial Pneumonitis (NSIP)
- • Cellular NSIP identical, fibrotic NSIP - honeycombing

Drug Toxicity
- • Identical findings, many drugs produce SLE pattern

Rheumatoid Arthritis
- • Interstitial thickening less common with SLE

Viral Pleuropericarditis
- • Identical appearance but limited course

Pathology

General
- • Collagen vascular disease involving
  - ○ Blood vessels: Pulmonary artery hypertension and vasculitis
  - ○ Serosa surfaces and joints
  - ○ Kidneys, CNS, skin
- • Etiology-pathogenesis

Systemic Lupus Erythematosus

- ○ Unknown
- ○ Drug-induced lupus 90% due to
    - ▪ Procainamide
    - ▪ Hydralazine
    - ▪ Isoniazid
    - ▪ Phenytoin
    - ▪ Thyroid blockers
    - ▪ Anti-arrhythmic drugs
    - ▪ Anticonvulsants
    - ▪ Antibiotics
- ○ Renal and CNS disease usually absent: Anti-DNA antibodies absent
- Epidemiology
    - ○ Women 10x men
    - ○ 50 cases per 100,000

Gross Pathologic-Surgical Features
- Pulmonary pathology nonspecific
    - ○ Vasculitis, hemorrhage, or BOOP

Microscopic Features
- Hematoxylin bodies pathognomonic but rare in lung (< 1%)

Clinical Issues

Presentation
- Diagnostic criteria (any four)
    - ○ Skin 80%: Malar rash; photosensitivity
    - ○ Oral ulceration 15%
    - ○ Arthropathy 85%
    - ○ Serositis (pericardial or pleural) 50%
    - ○ Renal proteinuria or casts 50%
    - ○ Neurologic epilepsy or psychosis 40%
    - ○ Hematologic anemia or pancytopenia
    - ○ Autoantibodies to DNA
- Pleural disease usually painful
- Hemorrhage may not result in hemoptysis
- Antiphospholipid antibodies in 40%
- Pulmonary function: Restrictive with normal diffusion capacity reflects diaphragm dysfunction
- Acute lupus pneumonitis
    - ○ Rare, life-threatening, immune complex disease
    - ○ Fever, cough, hypoxia requiring mechanical ventilation

Natural History
- Chronic disease (> 10 years) except in acute lupus pneumonitis
- At risk for thromboembolic disease, opportunistic infections

Treatment
- Steroids or immunosuppressants

Prognosis
- Chronic disease
- Acute lupus pneumonitis high mortality
- Most common cause of death sepsis or renal disease

Selected References
1. Fenlon HM et al: High-resolution chest CT in systemic lupus erythematosus. AJR 166:301-7, 1996
2. Wiedemann HP et al: Pulmonary manifestations of systemic lupus erythematosus. J Thorac Imaging 7:1-18, 1992

Diffuse Pulmonary Calcification

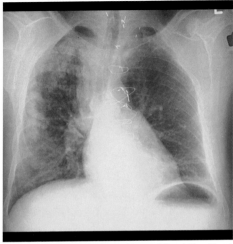

Moderate sized nodular opacities in the periphery of the right mid and upper lung, unchanged over 1 year. PO changes parathyroid surgery. Differential includes old granulomatous disease, diffuse pulmonary calcification, bronchoalveolar cell carcinoma, BOOP, and eosinophilic pneumonia.

Key Facts
- Metastatic pulmonary calcification
  - Metastatic pulmonary calcification secondary to hypercalcemia
  - Upper lobes most commonly affected (due to normal alkaline environment)
  - Mulberry-shaped, amorphous calcifications 3-10 mm diameter
- Alveolar microlithiasis
  - Alveolar microlithiasis familial
  - "Black" pleura sign due to subpleural cysts
  - Calcispherytes 0.01-3mm in diameter within alveoli
- Lung ossification
  - Benign finding most common in elderly men

Imaging Findings
General Features
- Best imaging clue: High density (or calcific) interstitial thickening
Chest Radiograph
- Normal high kVp technique not optimal for detection of calcification
- Metastatic pulmonary calcification
  - Upper lobes most commonly involved
  - Diffuse or focal, ill-defined, nodular and linear opacities
- Alveolar microlithiasis
  - Diffuse miliary calcifications "sandstorm"
  - "Black" pleura
  - Risk for spontaneous pneumothorax
- Lung ossification
  - Lower lobes dendritic or nodular calcifications 1-2 mm in diameter
CT Findings
- More sensitive than chest radiography for calcium
- Metastatic pulmonary calcification

Diffuse Pulmonary Calcification

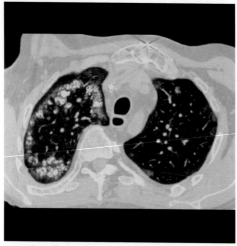

CT through upper lung (bone window). Lobulated nodular peripheral clusters are densely calcified. Diagnosis: Diffuse pulmonary calcification. Calcium preferentially deposits in the upper lung zones due to the more alkaline environment.

- o Mulberry-shaped amorphous calcification 3-10 mm in diameter
- o Vascular or soft-tissue calcification
- Alveolar microlithiasis
  - o Micronodular calcification preferentially peripheral and basilar
  - o Periphery secondary pulmonary lobule preferentially affected
  - o "Black" pleura represents subpleural cysts
- Lung ossification
  - o Dendritic or nodular 1-2 mm calcifications in periphery lower lobes
  - o May be associated with mild interstitial thickening

Bone Scanning
- All 3 conditions have uptake with bone seeking radionuclides

Imaging Recommendations
- CT or bone scanning sensitive for detection of calcium, CT useful to characterize distribution

Differential Diagnosis

Tuberculosis
- Upper lobes but doesn't have extensive calcification, cavitation not seen in metastatic calcification

Silicosis
- Nodules may calcify, occupational history important

Sarcoidosis
- Nodules may calcify, peribronchial distribution

Mitral Stenosis
- Left atrial enlargement and vascular redistribution, ossification primarily lower lobes

Amyloidosis
- Nodules larger, small nodules generally do not calcify

Diffuse Pulmonary Calcification

Pathology

<u>General</u>
- Metastatic calcification defined as calcium deposition in otherwise normal tissue
- Other than metastatic calcification, serum calcium usually normal in other conditions
- Genetics
  - Alveolar microlithiasis: Familial autosomal recessive (50%)
- Etiology-pathogenesis
  - Metastatic pulmonary calcification
    - Hypercalcemic conditions (high calcium phosphate product): Chronic renal failure, bone malignancies, hypervitaminosis D, diffuse myelomatosis, milk alkali syndrome, hyperparathyroidism
  - Physiology: Normally high V/Q ratio in upper lobes leads to alkaline pH (7.51), calcium less soluble in alkaline environment
  - Ossification and microlithiasis: Unknown

<u>Microscopic Features</u>
- Metastatic: Alveolar septal and vascular deposition
  - Alkaline tissues (stomach, kidney) also preferentially affected
- Microlithiasis: Calcispherytes (round concentrically laminated) in alveoli
  - Associated with fibrosis and pleural thickening
- Ossification: Branching mature bone within interstitium "coral tree"
- Ossification may occur in old fibrosis, usually incidental autopsy finding

Clinical Issues

<u>Presentation</u>
- Asymptomatic radiographic findings to slow, progressive respiratory failure
- 50% of patients with chronic renal failure have calcification at microscopic examination
- Lung ossification primarily seen in elderly men
- With severe disease, restrictive pulmonary function and decreased carbon monoxide diffusion in the lung (DLCO)

<u>Treatment</u>
- Correct hypercalcemia in metastatic calcification
- No known treatment for alveolar microlithiasis
- No treatment required for lung ossification

<u>Prognosis</u>
- Variable, from incidental finding (ossification) to death (microlithiasis)

Selected References
1. Hartman TE et al: Metastatic pulmonary calcification in patients with hypercalcemia: Findings on chest radiographs and CT scans. AJR 162:799-802, 1994
2. Brown K et al: Intrathoracic calcifications: Radiographic features and differential diagnoses. Radiographics 14:1247-61, 1994
3. Felson B et al: Idiopathic pulmonary ossification. Radiology 153:303-10, 1984

Diffuse Interstitial Pneumonias

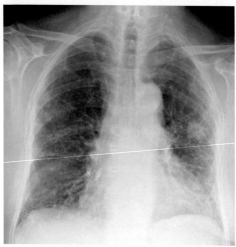

Usual Interstitial Pneumonia (UIP). Coarse diffuse peripheral interstitial thickening and honeycombing slightly worse in the lung bases. Heart is mildly enlarged. Cavitary mass mid left lung.

Key Facts
- Heterogeneous group of disorders of unknown cause
- Pathology: Patchy interstitial fibrosis and honeycombing
- Predominately peripheral and basilar
- Usual Interstitial Pneumonitis (UIP) most common of idiopathic interstitial pneumonias
- Prognosis poor

Imaging Findings
General Features
- Best imaging clue: Basilar peripheral honeycombing
Chest Radiograph
- General
  - Usually basilar and peripheral
  - Irregular linear opacities in contrast to the granulomatous diseases which are primarily nodular
  - Honeycombing and volume loss characteristic
  - Chest radiograph may be normal in spite of symptoms
- UIP (cryptogenic fibrosing alveolitis in UK)
  - Peripheral bilateral basilar irregular linear opacities
  - Volume loss, honeycombing in severe cases
  - ILO opacities: S, t, or u
- Acute Interstitial Pneumonia (AIP)
  - Synonym: Hamman-Rich syndrome
  - Diffuse pulmonary consolidation (not interstitial)
  - Intubated requiring mechanical ventilation
- Desquamative Interstitial Pneumonia (DIP)
  - Bilateral basilar irregular linear opacities admixed with consolidated lung 50%
  - Lung volumes preserved

Diffuse Interstitial Pneumonias

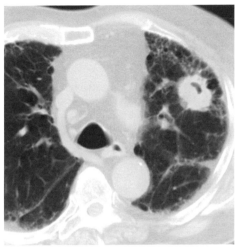

UIP and carcinoma of the lung. Central aspect of the lung is relatively spared. Periphery runs the gamut from normal to frank honeycombing. UIP often inhomogenous both in distribution and pattern. Cavitary mass was squamous cell carcinoma of the lung.

- o Honeycombing 10%
- Nonspecific Interstitial Pneumonitis (NSIP)
  - o Bibasilar irregular linear opacities; Slight decrease lung volumes

CT Findings
- General
  - o CT more sensitive than chest radiography
  - o Pattern and distribution, both useful in differential diagnosis
  - o Useful for mapping areas to biopsy
  - o Useful for prognosis; Ground-glass favorable, with honeycombing and traction bronchiectasis survival decreases
  - o CT may be normal in mild (or early) disease
- UIP
  - o Peripheral subpleural distribution 80%, honeycombing 95%
  - o Irregular linear opacities 80%, septal and intralobular thickening
  - o Ground-glass opacities 75%, traction bronchiectasis 50%
  - o Mediastinal nodes may be mildly enlarged (nodes < 2 cm diameter)
- DIP
  - o Symmetric ground-glass opacities, honeycombing unusual
  - o Lower lung zones predominance 70%, peripheral predominance 60%
  - o Irregular linear opacities, architectural distortion 50%, small cysts
  - o Traction bronchiectasis 30%
- NSIP
  - o Ground-glass opacities more common 100%, otherwise similar to UIP
  - o Bronchial dilatation of medium-sized bronchi more common than UIP
  - o Mediastinal adenopathy (<3 cm) 30%

Differential Diagnosis
Asbestosis
- Pleural plaques, subpleural fibrosis identical

Diffuse Interstitial Pneumonias

Drug Reaction
- Identical radiographic findings (bleomycin or nitrofurantoin)

Chronic Hypersensitivity Pneumonitis
- Not as severe at the extreme bases (last CT cut) which is usually the most severely involved with UIP

Sarcoidosis
- Nodular and peribronchial rather than reticular and subpleural

Bronchiolitis Obliterans Organizing Pneumonia (BOOP)
- Subpleural consolidation, no honeycombing

Pathology
General
- Unknown insult to alveolar wall and interstitium
- UIP thought to be repetitive insult vs. AIP as single overwhelming injury
- Etiology-pathogenesis: Unknown, speculation circulatory insult
  - DIP once thought to be cellular phase of UIP, now discredited

Gross Pathologic-Surgical Features
- Coarse honeycombing and volume loss
- Usually inhomogeneous both spatially and temporally
- AIP, DIP, and NSIP: Usually temporally homogeneous
- NSIP: Defined as those not fitting into other categories: Debatable whether this is a specific entity

Microscopic Features
- UIP: Predominately fibroblast proliferation
- AIP: Identical to DAD
- DIP: Intraalveolar accumulation of macrophages
- NSIP may be cellular or fibrotic

Clinical Issues
Presentation
- UIP and NSIP: Progressive dyspnea, dry cough and fatigue
- UIP: 5-7th decade, slight predominance in men
- AIP: Acute fever, cough, SOB rapidly progress to respiratory failure (days)
  - Diagnosis of exclusion, cultures negative, exclude drugs and toxins
- DIP: Smokers
- NSIP: 15% have collagen vascular disease, 15% exposure to noxious gas
- PFTs: Restrictive with decreased diffusion capacity

Natural History
- Intermittent episodes (UIP) to rapidly progressive (AIP)

Treatment
- Steroids, cytotoxic agents limited success
- Lung transplant

Prognosis
- Variable: UIP median survival 5 years, AIP mortality 80%, DIP mortality 25%, NSIP mortality 10%

Selected References
1. Hansell DM: Computed tomography of diffuse lung disease: Functional correlates. Eur Radiol 11:1666-1680, 2001
2. Hartman TE et al: Nonspecific interstitial pneumonia: Variable appearance at high-resolution chest CT. Radiology 217:701-5, 2000
3. Hartman TE et al: Disease progression in usual interstitial pneumonia compared with desquamative interstitial pneumonia. Assessment with serial CT. Chest 110:378-82, 1996

PocketRadiologist™
Chest
Top 100 Diagnoses

MEDIASTINUM

Thymoma

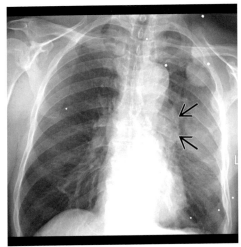

Malignant thymoma. Anterior mediastinal mass (arrows) with multiple drop metastases to the pleura of the left hemithorax.

Key Facts
- Most common anterior mediastinal mass
- May be calcified (rim or punctate) or cystic (generally larger tumors)
- 1/3 invasive, drop metastases to pleura
- Paraneoplastic syndromes (40%), myasthenia gravis (30%), pure red cell aplasia (5%), hypogammaglobulinemia (10%)

Imaging Findings
General Features
- Best imaging clue: Anterior mediastinal mass
Chest Radiograph
- Thymoma
  - Slow growing, lopsided, oval mass 5-10 cm in diameter
  - Centered over base of heart
  - Best seen lateral view, 60% subtle
  - Calcification 10%, rim or punctate
- Thymic hyperplasia
  - Anterior mediastinal mass, normal thymic shape
- Thymolipoma
  - Large anterior mediastinal mass
  - Often conforms to configuration of heart, mimics cardiomegaly
CT Findings
- Thymoma
  - Oval homogeneous mass
  - 1/3 calcification, rim or punctate
  - 1/3 cystic, generally larger tumors
  - Evaluate surrounding fat planes for invasion
  - Drop metastases to pleura
  - Transdiaphragmatic spread through aortic or esophageal hiatus
- Thymic hyperplasia

Thymoma

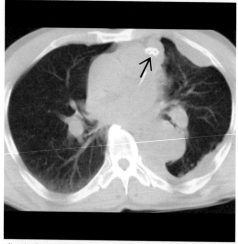

Anterior mediastinal mass is partially calcified (arrow). Multiple discreet pleural metastases in left hemithorax. In thymoma, calcification is not a sign of benignancy.

- ○ Gland normal shape but larger than normal
- ○ Homogeneous, no calcification or cysts
- • Thymolipoma
  - ○ Fatty mass interspersed with strands and islands of soft tissue
  - ○ Proportion of fat and soft tissue either equal or predominately fat

<u>MRI Findings</u>
- • Thymoma
  - ○ No advantage over CT
  - ○ Decreased T1, increased T2
  - ○ Invasive tumors may have multinodular appearance

<u>Imaging Recommendations</u>
- • CT utility detect subtle tumors, characterize anterior mediastinal masses

Differential Diagnosis

<u>Germ Cell Tumor</u>
- • Younger patients, tumor often more inhomogeneous

<u>Lymphoma</u>
- • Multiple nodal masses, involvement other lymph node groups, spleen maybe enlarged

<u>Metastases</u>
- • Known GU or head and neck malignancy, no calcification

<u>Thyroid Goiter</u>
- • Higher attenuation (due to iodine), connected to thyroid gland

<u>Lipomatosis</u>
- • Diffuse fat density, steroid use

<u>Liposarcoma</u>
- • Soft tissue predominates over fat density

Thymoma

Pathology
General
- Normal gland not lobulated, role T cell maturation
  - 2 lobes joined superiorly, left lobe larger than right
  - Normal fatty involution with age
- Age < 20: Maximal thickness < 1.8 cm
- Age > 20: Maximal thickness < 1.3 cm
- Embryology-anatomy
  - Origin: 3rd & 4th brachial cleft (absence: DiGeorge syndrome)
- Etiology-pathogenesis
  - Hyperplasia: Normal thymus involutes with stress, steroids, or chemotherapy, will regrow with removal of the insult, sometimes growing larger than the initial size of the gland (thymic rebound)

Gross Pathologic-Surgical Features
- Invasive thymoma not histologic diagnosis
- Thymolipoma: Large, encapsulated tumors

Microscopic Features
- Thymoma: Epithelial or lymphocytic, 1/3 invasive
- Hyperplasia: True hyperplasia of cortex and medulla
- Thymolipoma: Normal thymic tissue admixed with normal fat

Staging Criteria Thymoma
- Stage I: Intact capsule
- Stage II: Microscopic capsular invasion
- Stage III: Invades surrounding structures
- Stage IV: (a): Pleural drop metastases; (b): Distant metastases

Clinical Issues
Presentation
- Thymoma
  - 15% all mediastinal masses, 50% anterior mediastinal masses
  - Age 50, M=F
  - 50% nonspecific symptoms
  - Paraneoplastic syndromes (40%):
    - Myasthenia gravis (30%); thymoma in myasthenia gravis (15%)
    - Pure red cell aplasia (5%); thymoma in red cell aplasia (50%)
    - Hypogammaglobulinemia (10%); thymoma in hypogammaglobulinemia (5%)
  - Other associated malignances: Lung, lymphoma, thyroid
- Thymic hyperplasia
  - Causes: Post chemotherapy (10%), chronic adrenal insufficiency, thyrotoxicosis, myasthenia gravis
  - Develops a few months post therapy, mistaken for recurrent disease
- Thymolipoma
  - No association with myasthenia gravis
  - Young (mean age 25), no gender preference

Treatment
- Thymoma: Surgery, radiation and chemotherapy invasive disease
- No therapy for thymic hyperplasia

Selected References
1. Morgenthaler TI et al: Thymoma. Mayo Clin Proc 68:1110-23, 1993
2. Rosado-de-Christenson ML et al: Thymoma: Radiologic-pathologic correlation. Radiographics 12:151-68, 1992

Mediastinal Germ Cell Tumor

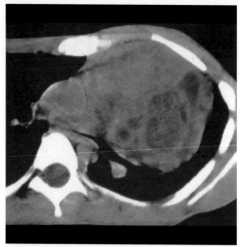

Klinefelter's syndrome. Noncontrast CT. Large anterior heterogenous mediastinal mass displaying soft tissue and fat attenuation. No calcificaiton.

Key Facts
- Teratoma, seminomas, nonseminomas (embryonal cell, endodermal sinus, choriocarcinoma, mixed germ cell tumor)
- 10% of anterior mediastinal tumors
- Spectrum: Solid, cystic, or necrotic tumors, benign tumors may have calcification
- Mature teratomas CT: Lobulated multilocular tumors, 25% have calcification
- Seminoma CT: Homogeneous midline tumors
- Nonseminomas: Irregular with large, central, low-attenuation, septated component

Imaging Findings
General Features
- Best imaging clue: Large, anterior mediastinal mass
Chest Radiograph
- Teratoma
  - Lopsided, round, sharply-marginated, anterior mediastinal mass
  - 25% calcify
  - Centered over PA, mimics PA stenosis (even murmur on physical exam)
- Seminoma
  - Bulky, lobulated, anterior mediastinal mass straddles midline
  - Calcification rare
- Nonseminomas
  - Large, irregular-shaped, anterior mediastinal mass
  - Pleural effusions common
  - Pulmonary metastases common
CT Findings
- Teratoma
  - Multiloculated mass with variable thickness walls

Mediastinal Germ Cell Tumor

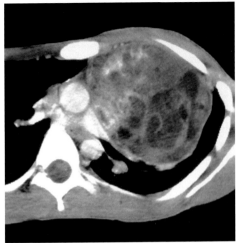

Portions of mass enhance with intravenous contrast. Mass is centered over and compresses the main pulmonary artery. Diagnosis: Malignant germ cell tumor. Location of mass is typical, and may mimic pulmonary artery stenosis, even producing the murmur of stenosis

- o May contain fat, calcification, fluid, soft tissue
- o Septa and rim may enhance with contrast
- Seminoma
  - o Lobulated homogeneous mass
  - o Calcification rare
  - o May metastasize to regional lymph nodes, bone
- Nonseminomas
  - o Large, irregular-shaped mass with ill-defined margins
  - o More than 50% central low attenuation
  - o Obliterates adjacent fat planes
  - o Pleural and pericardial effusions common
  - o Pulmonary metastases

Imaging Recommendations
- CT recommended to evaluate extent and characterize mediastinal mass

Differential Diagnosis
Thymoma
- Thymoma associated with paraneoplastic syndromes

Lymphoma
- Lymphoma rarely calcifies before treatment

Carcinoid
- Rarely calcifies, osteoblastic bone metastases, paraneoplastic syndrome

Pathology
General
- Derived from all 3 cell lines or embryologic cell rests

Gross Pathologic-Surgical Features
- Large bulky tumors often heterogeneous with cysts, necrosis or solid components including bone

Mediastinal Germ Cell Tumor

Microscopic Features
- Teratoma
  - Primitive organ formation
    - Teeth, skin, hair, bone, cartilage, pancreatic tissue
    - Spectrum: Mature (solid), cystic (dermoid), immature fetal (teratocarcinoma)
- Seminoma
  - Uniform sheets of round cells admixed with lymphocytes
- Nonseminomas
  - Embryonal: Large malignant cells arranged in sheets
  - Endodermal: Glandular cords of neoplastic cells
  - Choriocarcinoma: Large, round, multinucleated cells (syncytiotrophoblastic); hemorrhage

Clinical Issues
Presentation
- Teratoma
  - 60% of germ cell tumors
  - Age 20-30, M=F
  - Most asymptomatic
  - Digestive enzymes may burrow into lung or bronchus
    - Trichoptysis (hair expectoration)
- Seminoma (germinoma, dysgerminoma)
  - 30% of germ cell tumors
  - Age 30-40, M > F
  - Usually symptomatic
  - Elevated beta HCG
- Nonseminomas
  - 10% of germ cell tumors
  - Age 30-40, M > F
  - Most symptomatic
  - Associated with hematologic malignancies
  - 20% Klinefelter's syndrome (gynecomastia, testicular atrophy, increased FSH)

Treatment
- Teratoma: Surgery
- Seminoma: Radiation
- Nonseminomas: Chemotherapy and surgery

Prognosis
- Variable, excellent benign tumors, poor for metastatic disease

Selected References
1. Choi SJ et al: Mediastinal teratoma: CT differentiation of ruptured and unruptured tumors. AJR 171:591-4, 1998
2. Strollo DC et al: Primary mediastinal tumors: Part I. Tumors of the anterior mediastinum. Chest 112:511-22, 1997
3. Rosado-de-Christenson ML et al: From the archives of the AFIP. Mediastinal germ cell tumors: Radiologic and pathologic correlation. Radiographics 12:1013-30, 1992

Lymphoma

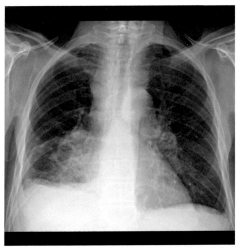

Non-Hodgkin's lymphoma. Diffuse mediastinal widening and right hilar adenopathy. Bilateral pleural effusions, right greater than left.

Key Facts
- Hodgkin's preferentially involves anterior superior mediastinum
- Non-Hodgkin's equally involves any mediastinal nodal group
- Nodes may calcify post treatment (rim or mulberry)
- Non-Hodgkin's may spontaneously regress
- Posttransplanatation lymphoproliferative disorder (PTLD) Epstein-Barr virus related

Imaging Findings
Chest Radiograph
- Hodgkin's lymphoma
  - Initially, 85% intrathoracic involvement
  - Most commonly involves anterior superior mediastinal nodes
    - Nodes rarely calcify before treatment: 5% post therapy: Rim or Multiple discrete deposits (mulberry)
    - Pericardial fat pad sign: Enlargement of pericardial lymph nodes; Pericardial nodes undertreated due to cardiac lead blockers to protect heart from radiation therapy
  - Lung
    - 10% at presentation, almost always in conjunction with nodes
    - Multiple pulmonary nodules or multifocal consolidation
  - Pleural effusion (15%)
- Non-Hodgkin's lymphoma
  - Initially, 50% intrathoracic involvement
  - Anterior and posterior nodes equally likely except lymphoblastic and large B-cell lymphoma primarily involve anterior mediastinum
  - Lung
    - Multiple pulmonary nodules may cavitate
    - Lymphomatoid granulomatosis triad: CNS – skin – lung
    - Airspace mass (solitary or multiple, includes pseudolymphoma)
    - Diffuse reticular thickening (lymphocytic interstitial pneumonia)

Lymphoma

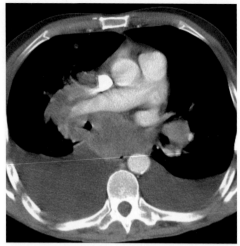

Non-Hodgkin's lymphoma. Multiple lymph nodes enlarged including both hila and subcarinal regions. Moderated to large bilateral pleural effusions.

- ○ Pleura: Effusions or focal pleural mass
- PTLD
  - ○ Nodules: Peripheral and basilar, no air-bronchograms, rarely cavitate
  - ○ Focal consolidation: Bronchiolitis obliterans organizing pneumonia (BOOP) like
  - ○ Hilar and mediastinal adenopathy

<u>CT Findings</u>
- Hodgkin's lymphoma
  - ○ Nodes minimally enhance, 1/3 nodes cystic or necrotic
  - ○ Thymic cysts may develop prior to or following treatment

Differential Diagnosis
<u>Germ Cell Tumor</u>
- Patients younger, tumor inhomogeneous

<u>Thymoma</u>
- May have calcification (rare in lymphoma prior to treatment)

<u>Metastases</u>
- History of GU or head and neck tumors

<u>Thyroid Goiter</u>
- Tumor higher attenuation, connected to thyroid gland

<u>Sarcoid</u>
- Nodes symmetric, uniform in size

<u>Tuberculosis</u>
- Rim enhancing nodes

Pathology
<u>General</u>
- Minimal mass effect (not obstructive) compared to carcinoma
- Etiology-pathogenesis
  - ○ PTLD: Cyclosporine inhibits suppressor T cells allowing unrestricted proliferation of EB virus infected B-cells

Lymphoma

Microscopic Features
- Hodgkin's: Reed Sternberg cell
- Non-Hodgkin's: Clonal proliferation either of T and B cell origin
- PTLD: Spectrum benign polyclonal to malignant monoclonal, most B-cell

Staging or Grading Criteria
- Hodgkin's: Nodular sclerosis (70%); mixed cellularity (20%); lymphocytic predominant (5%); lymphocytic deplete (5%)
- Non-Hodgkin's (Low – intermediate – high grade)
  - Small (lymphocytic or non-cleaved cell), immunoblastic
  - Follicular (small cleaved, mixed, or large cell)
  - Diffuse (small cleaved, mixed, large cell), lymphoblastic

Clinical Issues

Presentation
- Hodgkin's
  - Bimodal peak 3rd & 5th decade, M > F
    - Stage I: Single lymph node group
    - Stage II: 2 lymph node groups same side of diaphragm
    - Stage III: Nodes on both sides of diaphragm
    - Stage IV: Extranodal sites
    - A: Asymptomatic
    - B: Symptoms (20%) fever, night sweats, weight loss of 10%
- Non-Hodgkins
  - Any age, peak 55
  - Higher risk
    - Immunodeficiency: Post-transplant, AIDS, Wiskott-Aldrich, ataxia-telangiectasia, Sjögen's syndrome (LIP)
    - Epstein-Barr virus: Burkitt's, cyclosporine induced PTLD
  - Usually extensive disease at diagnosis, staging same as for Hodgkins
- Post-transplant lymphoproliferative disorder
  - Incidence 5% solid organ transplants, children more susceptible
  - Usually develops in 1st year post-transplant (peak 3-4 months)
  - Other common sites: GI, oropharynx, cervical lymph nodes
  - Asymptomatic to influenza symptoms (fever, pharyngitis, cervical lymphadenopathy)

Treatment
- Hodgkin's: Mantle radiation therapy, chemotherapy, BMT
- Non-Hodgkin's: Surveillance for low-grade asymptomatic patients
  - Radiation therapy, chemotherapy, and bone marrow transplantation
  - May spontaneously regress
- PTLD: decrease cyclosporine dose

Prognosis
- Hodgkin's: Good, 90% cure
  - 2nd tumors: AML, Non-Hodgkin's
- Non-Hodgkin's: Depends on bulk and histopathologic diagnosis
- Low-grade tumors may evolve to higher grade

Selected References
1. Collins J et al: Epstein-Barr-virus-associated lymphoproliferative disease of the lung: CT and histologic findings. Radiology 208:749-59, 1998
2. Strollo DC et al: Primary mediastinal tumors: Part II. Tumors of the middle and posterior mediastinum. Chest 112:1344-57, 1997
3. Castellino RA et al: Hodgkin disease: Contributions of chest CT in the initial staging evaluation. Radiology 160:603-5, 1986

Lymphoproliferative Disorders

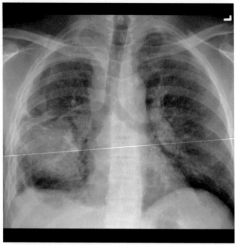

Angioimmunoblastic lymphadenopathy. Hilar and mediasitnal adenopathy. Large homogenoeous opacity right base. Pleural effusion or thickening right hemithorax.

Key Facts
- Spectrum of lymphoid disorders that range from benign to low-grade malignancies
- Angioimmunoblastic lymphadenopathy may be secondary to Dilantin
- Castleman's disease lymph nodes may show vascular enhancement
- Post-transplant lymphoproliferative disorder related to EB virus

Imaging Findings
Chest Radiograph
- Plasma cell granuloma
  - Solitary lung mass, sharply marginated 1–10 cm diameter
  - Usually lower lobe, calcification and cavitation uncommon
  - No pleural effusion or adenopathy
- Castleman's disease (angiofollicular hyperplasia)
  - Localized: Solitary mediastinal mass
  - Diffuse: Multiple nodes, occasionally interstitial thickening lung
- Pseudolymphoma
  - Large, consolidated mass with ill-defined margin (due to lymphatic extension surrounding lung)
- Lymphocytic interstitial pneumonia (LIP)
  - Diffuse interstitial thickening, predominately basilar
  - Adenopathy or pleural effusions rare
- Post-transplant lymphoproliferative disorders (PTLD)
  - Multiple pulmonary nodules with or without adenopathy
- Angioimmunoblastic lymphadenopathy
  - Hilar mediastinal adenopathy with nonspecific interstitial or alveolar opacities in the lung
  - Hepatosplenomegaly
CT Findings
- Castleman's or angioimmunoblastic lymphadenopathy lymph nodes may enhance, Castleman's may occasionally calcify

142

Lymphoproliferative Disorders

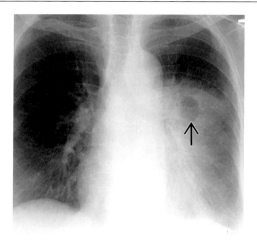

Pseudolymphoma. Focal mass like area of consolidation has slowly grown over 11 years. Consolidation contains cyst or cavity (arrow).

- LIP: Centrilobular nodules, occasional thin-walled cystic lesions, lymph nodes may be enlarged (not demonstrated at chest radiography)
- PTLD: Nodules may have low-density centers and occasionally demonstrate halo sign, usually located along peribronchovascular or subpleural areas

Imaging Recommendations
- CT useful to characterize both lung and degree of mediastinal adenopathy

Differential Diagnosis
- None

Pathology
General
- Bronchus associated lymphoid tissue (BALT) extends from nodal clusters in airway bifurcations to lymphocyte clusters at proximity of lymphatics in respiratory bronchiole
  - BALT extensive, positioned to handle large number of inhaled or circulating antigens
  - Polyclonal proliferation consistent with benign disease, monoclonal proliferation of lymphocytes consistent with lymphoma. Clonal groups determined by special stains
- Etiology-pathogenesis
  - PTLD: Related to EB infection, immunosuppression with cyclosporine allows unrestricted proliferation of EB virus infected cells, may become monoclonal and malignant
  - Angioimmunoblastic lymphadenopathy: Possible hypersensitive reaction, associated with drug reactions (Dilantin, insulin, penicillin)
- Epidemiology
  - PTLD: Prevalence 5%, highest in lung transplants
  - LIP: Associated with Sjögren's syndrome or AIDS

Lymphoproliferative Disorders

<u>Microscopic Features</u>
- Plasma cell granuloma: Admixture plasma cells, lymphocytes and histiocytes
- Castleman's disease: Localized (90% - hyaline vascular type), Diffuse (10% - plasma cell type)
- Pseudolymphoma and LIP identical: Small lymphocytes and plasma cells, occasional fibrosis
- PTLD and angioimmunoblastic lymphadenopathy: Proliferation of immunoblasts

Clinical Issues
<u>Presentation</u>
- Plasma cell granuloma: Most common lung mass in children, usually asymptomatic or nonspecific cough, fever, chest pain; no relationship to multiple myeloma
- Castleman's disease: Localized usually asymptomatic, diffuse symptomatic – weight loss, fever both in patients < 30
- Pseudolymphoma: Asymptomatic middle-aged adults
- PTLD: Time between transplant and disease varies from 1 month to years; nonspecific symptoms
- Angioimmunoblastic lymphadenopathy: Older adults, rapid progression with rash and pruritus, anemia and dysproteinemia common
- LIP: Cough, dyspnea and dysgammaglobulinemia, age varies

<u>Treatment</u>
- Varies with disease from observation, resection, to chemotherapy for lymphomas
- PTLD: Decrease cyclosporine dosage

<u>Prognosis</u>
- Castleman's: Localized good prognosis, diffuse poorer prognosis
- Plasma cell granuloma: Good prognosis
- Angioimmunoblastic lymphadenopathy, PTLD: Variable
- Prognosis also depends on evolution to frank lymphoma

Selected References
1. McAdams HP et al: Castleman disease of the thorax: Radiologic features with clinical and histopathologic correlation. Radiology 209:221-8, 1998
2. Collins J et al: Epstein-Barr-virus-associated lymphoproliferative disease of the lung: CT and histologic findings. Radiology 208:749-59, 1998
3. Bragg DG et al: Lymphoproliferative disorders of the lung: Histopathology, clinical manifestations, and imaging features. AJR 163:273-81, 1994

Superior Vena Caval Obstruction

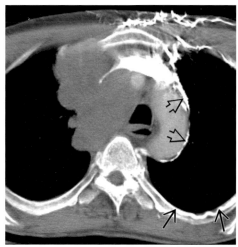

Superior Vena Cava (SVC) Obstruction. Bronchogenic carcinoma extending into mediastinum narrowing left brachiocephalic vein and obstructing SVC. Collaterals: Chest wall, intercostals (arrows), and left superior intercostals vein (open arrow).

Key Facts
- Most common cause of SVC obstruction: Bronchogenic carcinoma
- Mediastinal widening and dilated azygos vein and aortic nipple clues to SVC obstruction on the chest radiograph
- CT ideal examination to demonstrate cause of obstruction, location and collateral vessels
- Periscapular collaterals may be seen in normal patients

Imaging Findings
General Features
- Best imaging clue: Mediastinal widening with enlarged azygos vein and aortic nipple

Chest Radiograph
- Mediastinal widening, nonspecific
- Venous collaterals
  - Large azygos vein
  - Dilated left superior intercostal vein (aortic nipple)

CT Findings
- Narrowing or obstruction of SVC
- Visualization of collateral pathways
  - Azygos – hemiazygos system
  - Vertebral venous plexus
  - Internal mammary veins
  - Periscapular
  - Intercostal
  - Internal thoracic vein
  - Lateral thoracic system
    - Pathway to epigastric veins to periumbilical veins to left portal vein
    - Focal contrast enhancement of liver parenchyma adjacent to falciform ligament

Superior Vena Caval Obstruction

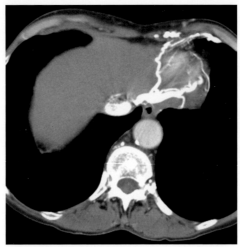

SVC obstruction. Peridiaphragmatic venous collaterals draining into IVC. Diagnosis of SVC obstruction requires the visualization of collateral vessels.

<u>MRI Findings</u>
- Similar to CT, does not require contrast administration
- Poor demonstration of calcification

<u>Imaging Recommendations</u>
- CT recommended to determine cause of obstruction and define venous anatomy

Differential Diagnosis

<u>Pseudocollaterals</u>
- Hyperabduction of arm may narrow subclavian vein normally, contrast injection may then opacify periscapular veins normally

<u>Interruption of the Inferior Vena Cava with Azygos Continuation</u>
- No collaterals, no obstructing mass

Pathology

<u>General</u>
- Major collateral pathways between SVC and IVC
  - Azygos-hemiazygos veins
  - Vertebral venous system
  - Internal mammary veins
  - Lateral thoracic system
    - Lateral thoracic vein
    - Thoracoepigastric and superficial epigastric veins
    - Blood shunted to periumbilical veins and the left portal vein along falciform ligament
- Epidemiology
  - 80% malignant neoplasms, 20% benign
  - Causes
    - Bronchogenic carcinoma
    - Metastases, especially breast
    - Lymphoma

Superior Vena Caval Obstruction

- Fibrosing mediastinitis
- Radiation
- Venous catheters or pacemaker wire induced thrombosis

Gross Pathologic-Surgical Features
- Whether malignant or benign, obstructing mass is usually not resectable

Microscopic Features
- No specific features

Clinical Issues

Presentation
- Asymptomatic to dyspnea, choking, neurologic impairment
- Symptoms depend on time course, slowly developing obstruction allows time for collateral development with few or no symptoms
- Neck vein distention and edema upper torso with acute SVC obstruction

Treatment
- Venous stents
- Radiation therapy for malignant lesions
- Anticoagulation for thrombosis
- Surgical bypass difficult, rarely performed

Prognosis
- Depends on cause

Selected References
1. Standford W et al: Superior vena cava obstruction: A venographic classification. AJR 148: 259-62, 1987
2. Gosselin MV et al: Altered intravascular contrast material flow dynamics: Clues for refining thoracic CT diagnosis. AJR 169:1597-603, 1997

Extramedullary Hematopoiesis

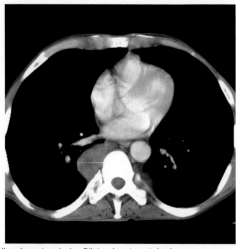

Extramedullary hematopoiesis. Bilateral costovertebral masses are usually centered on vertebral bodies. Masses are sharply defined and maybe slightly lobulated.

Key Facts
- Rare due to marrow expansion in severe anemias: Thalassemia, hemolytic anemias, sickle cell disease
- Asymptomatic
- Posterior mediastinal mass, unilateral or bilateral usually between T8–T12
- Bone changes: Marrow expansion, trabecular prominence
- May contain fat at CT
- May enhance at CT

Imaging Findings
General Features
- Best imaging clue: Multiple lobulated posterior mediastinal masses with vertebral bodies which have prominent trabeculae

Chest Radiograph
- Posterior mediastinal mass
  - Unilateral or bilateral
  - Located anywhere along spine, most common between T8–T12
  - Sharply demarcated, lobulated, centered on vertebral bodies
- Bone changes
  - Marrow expansion
  - Prominent trabeculae
  - Bones may be normal
- Subcostal rib masses may also be found
- As blood forming organs: Hepatosplenomegaly may also be found
  - Spleen, however, will be small in sickle cell disease

CT Findings
- May contain fat
- Calcification absent
- Will enhance with contrast administration
- No bone erosion

Extramedullary Hematopoiesis

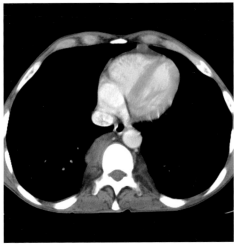

Extramedullary hematopoiesis. Location generally lower thoracic spine. No bone erosion. Masses may enhance with contrast administration.

- Size 5 mm to > 5 cm
- Very slow growth
- Most common location along costovertebral junction

Nuclear Medicine Findings
- Uptake Tc ^{99m} sulfur colloid
- Radionuclide scans may be normal

Imaging Recommendations
- CT in patient with appropriate history usually sufficient for diagnosis

Differential Diagnosis

Neurofibromas
- May be multiple, however usually discrete, different from the long mass of extramedullary hematopiesis, pressure erosion on adjacent vertebral body, no marrow expansion

Paragangliomas
- Intense enhancement with contrast, extramedullary hematopoiesis has mottled enhancement, no marrow expansion

Esophageal Varices
- Multiple small vessels enhance, no marrow expansion

Pathology

General
- Benign marrow elements outside the marrow in patients with severe anemia
- Etiology-pathogenesis
  - Extrusion of marrow through cortical defects or
  - Growth of heterotopic or multipotential cells

Gross Pathologic-Surgical Features
- Lobulated masses of hematopoietic marrow

149

Extramedullary Hematopoiesis

Clinical Issues

Presentation
- Asymptomatic
  - No treatment required
- Rarely cause cord compression

Treatment
- Responds to small doses of radiation if cord compression

Prognosis
- Related to anemia

Selected References
1. Papavasiliou C et al: The marrow heterotopia in thalassemia. Eur J Radiol 6:92-6, 1986
2. Korsten J et al: Extramedullary hematopoiesis in patients with thalassemia anemia. Radiology 95:257-63, 1970

Cystic Foregut Malformations

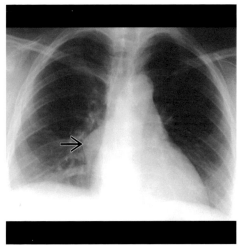

Asymptomatic patient. Right sided mediastinal mass (arrow). Margins are sharp. Differential must include vascular aneurysms and other possibilities: Bronchogenic cyst, pericardial cyst, adenopathy, pleural or lung mass.

Key Facts
- 10% of all mediastinal masses
- Congenital budding abnormalities from the foregut or notochord
- Usually asymptomatic
- Round sharply-marginated mass
- Thin-walled cystic structures at CT
- Esophageal and neurenteric cysts tubular
- Cysts with gastric or pancreatic tissue may hemorrhage or ulcerate

Imaging Findings
General Features
- Best imaging clue: Thin-walled subcarinal cyst at CT
Chest Radiograph
- Round, sharply-marginated mass 2-10 cm in size
- Middle mediastinal locations: Right paratracheal or subcarinal region
  - Can occur anywhere in mediastinum
  - 10% in lung
- Esophageal and neurenteric cysts more tubular, oriented vertically along esophagus and spine
CT Findings
- Bronchogenic cyst
  - Thin-walled
  - Cyst, variable attenuation
    - Low to high (blood, calcium, or protein)
  - Moldable, rarely cause obstruction
  - No contrast enhancement
- Esophageal duplication cyst
  - Right sided
  - Adjacent to esophagus

Cystic Foregut Malformations

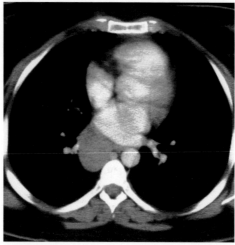

CT. Sharply marginated homogenous low density mass in the azygoesophageal recess. Diagnosis: Bronchogenic cyst.

- o Tubular vertical shape
- o May ulcerate into esophagus or airway (air-fluid level)
- Neurenteric cyst
  - o Right sided
  - o Posterior mediastinum
  - o Long vertical lesion
  - o Associated with vertebral anomalies
    - Hemivertebra
    - Sagittal clefts
  - o Vertebral anomalies superior to cyst
  - o Most commonly located upper thoracic spine

MRI Findings
- If CT indeterminate for cyst, MRI may demonstrate cystic nature of mass
- Variable signal intensity T1 due to fluid and protein
- High signal intensity T2

Imaging Recommendations
- CT procedure of choice to characterize mediastinal masses

Differential Diagnosis
Lymphoma
- Multiple nodal masses not cystic
Bronchogenic Carcinoma
- Older smoker, if cyst wall nodular and thick consider carcinoma
Nerve Sheath Tumors or Sympathetic Ganglion Tumors
- Not generally cystic

Pathology
General
- Cysts with muscular or fibrous walls with a lining of bronchial or enteric epithelium
- Embryology-anatomy

Cystic Foregut Malformations

- o Congenital abnormal budding from ventral foregut
- o Notochord adjacent to foregut and may give rise to neurenteric cysts
- o Early duplication
  - ▪ Mediastinal
- o Late duplication
  - ▪ Lung location
  - ▪ 10% of all bronchogenic cysts

Gross Pathologic-Surgical Features
- • Unilocular cyst containing mucus, watery fluid, or purulent material

Microscopic Features
- • Bronchogenic cyst
  - o Lined with respiratory epithelium, contain cartilage
- • Esophageal duplication cyst
  - o Contain gastric mucosa or pancreatic tissue
    - ▪ More likely to ulcerate or hemorrhage
- • Neurenteric cyst
  - o Admixture of gastric and neural tissue elements

Clinical Issues

Presentation
- • 10% all mediastinal masses
- • Accidentally discovered in young adults < 35
- • Usually asymptomatic
- • Chest pain, cough, wheezing

Treatment
- • Surgical resection for symptomatic lesions
- • Needle aspiration
- • Observation

Prognosis
- • Cure with surgical removal

Selected References
1. Strollo DC et al: Primary mediastinal tumors: Part II. Tumors of the middle and posterior mediastinum. Chest 112:1344-57, 1997
2. Panicek DM et al: The continuum of pulmonary developmental anomalies. Radiographics 7:747-72, 1987

Pulmonary Sequestration

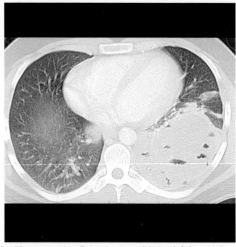

Young adult with pneumonia. Extensive consolidation left lower lobe with multiple air-fluid levels. Air-fluid levels either due to necrotizing pneumonia or involvement of otherwise abnormal cystic lung.

Key Facts
- Left-sided inferior paraspinal mass
- Single or multiple cysts common and may be air filled
- Systemic artery from aorta seen in 80% at CT
- Lung bordering sequestration maybe hyperinflated
- Lung tissue: No bronchial communication, systemic arterial supply
- Intralobar 75%, maybe congenital or acquired
- Extralobar usually associated with other anomalies, earlier presentation
- Surgical removal for chronic infection or hemoptysis

Imaging Findings
General Features
- Best imaging clue: Chronic left-sided inferior paraspinal mass
Chest Radiograph
- Inferior paraspinal mass or opacity
- Margins sharp or ill-defined
- Contour smooth to irregular
- 1/3 contain air or air-fluid level
- "Chronic pneumonia"
  - May decrease in size with antibiotic therapy
- Pleural effusion rare
- Intralobar location: Left sided (60%)
- Extralobar location: Left sided (80%)
CT Findings
- Complex lesion containing solid, fluid, and cystic components
- 80% systemic arterial supply demonstrated from aorta
- Cysts single or multiple
- Border with normal lung may contain emphysematous or hyperinflated lung
- Heterogeneous contrast enhancement

Pulmonary Sequestration

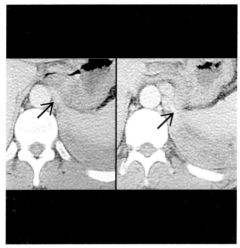

Pulmonary sequestration. Contiguous images after administration of contrast, arterial supply from the descending aorta courses to the sequestered lung (arrows). Arterial supply often courses through the inferior pulmonary ligament.

- May contain calcification

Angiography Findings
- Identify feeding artery
  - Thoracic aorta 75%
  - Abdominal aorta 20%
  - Intercostal artery 5%
  - May be single or multiple
  - Feeding artery may also supply normal lung
- Use has decreased with CT
  - Lack of identification at CT usually due to multiple small arteries

Differential Diagnosis

Neurogenic Tumor
- Usually not cystic, no feeding artery

Pleural Tumor
- Not heterogeneous, no feeding artery

Lung Cancer
- Grows, no feeding artery

Pneumonia
- No feeding artery, will evolve with therapy

Abscess
- No feeding artery

Pathology

General
- Intralobar
  - 75% all sequestrations
  - No separate pleural investment
  - Artery from aorta

Pulmonary Sequestration

- Usually enters lung through inferior pulmonary ligament
  - o Venous drainage: Pulmonary vein
  - o Foregut communication: Rare
  - o Associated anomalies: Rare
    - Esophagobronchial fistula
    - Bronchogenic cyst
    - Cystic adenomatoid malformation
- Extralobar
  - o 25% all sequestrations
  - o Separate pleural investment
  - o Artery from pulmonary or small systemic vessel
  - o Venous drainage: Azygos, hemiazygos
  - o Foregut communication: More common
  - o Associated anomalies: Common
- Etiology-pathogenesis
  - o Congenital or acquired inflammatory lesions

<u>Microscopic Features</u>
- Chronic inflammation, cysts and fibrosis
- No communication with bronchi
- Atherosclerotic changes in arterial supply common even in the young

Clinical Issues

<u>Presentation</u>
- Intralobar
  - o Equal gender
- Extralobar
  - o More common males
  - o Neonates, other anomalies often lethal
- Asymptomatic, incidentally discovered (20%)
- Chronic cough, recurrent pneumonia, hemoptysis, chest pain
  - o Hemoptysis may be life-threatening
- CHF in infants

<u>Treatment</u>
- Surgical resection for symptomatic lesions

Selected References
1. Frazier AA et al: Intralobar sequestration: Radiologic-pathologic correlation. Radiographics 17:725-45, 1997
2. Panicek DM et al: The continuum of pulmonary developmental anomalies. Radiographics 7:747-72, 1987
3. Savic B et al: Lung sequestration: Report of seven cases and review of 540 published cases. Thorax 34:96-101, 1979

Diaphragm Hernias

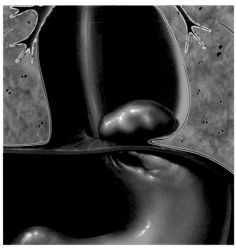

Paraesophageal hernia. The esophagogastric junction remains in the normal position while the fundus herniates through the hiatus.

Key Facts
- Hiatal hernia common incidental retrocardiac mass
- Suspect gastric ulcer in hiatal hernia with new unexplained pleural effusion
- Congenital diaphragmatic hernia cause of neonatal respiratory distress
- Gastric volvulus – double air-fluid level above and below diaphragm
- Morgagni hernia: Anterior, usually right sided
- Bochdalek hernia: Posterior, usually left sided
- Adult hernias usually asymptomatic
- Complications: Reflux, ulceration, bleeding, stricture

Imaging Findings
<u>General Features</u>
- Best imaging clue: Intrathoracic air-containing mass adjacent to diaphragm

<u>Chest Radiograph</u>
- Sliding hiatal hernia
  - Smooth hemispherical retrocardiac mass
  - Usually contain air or air-fluid level
  - Pleural effusion
    - New unexplained pleural effusion, suspect gastric ulcer in hernia sac
- Paraesophageal hernia
  - Gastric volvulus
    - Double air-fluid level above (retrocardiac) and below diaphragm (normal left subdiaphragmatic location)
    - Organoaxial rotation
    - Efferent loop may obstruct
- Morgagni
  - Right anterior paracardiac mass
  - May contain bowel

Diaphragm Hernias

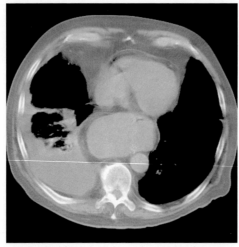

Hiatal hernia. Large fluid filled stomach may be mistaken for a mass. Note small collection of air. Moderate sized right pleural effusion. For unexplained effusion, consideration should be given to an ulcer in the intrathoracic portion of the stomach.

- Bochdalek
  - Posterolateral diaphragm
  - Congenital
    - 85% left sided
    - Contain fat, bowel, spleen
    - Contralateral mediastinal shift

Esophogram Findings
- Useful to determine anatomy and motility
- Mucosal complications, esophagitis, ulcers and strictures

CT Findings
- Sliding hernia: Complex mass with soft tissue, fat, air, and oral contrast
- Morgagni: Usually contain fat only
- Bochdalek: Usually contain fat, occasionally kidney or bowel

Imaging Recommendations
- Hiatal hernia chest radiograph, occasionally esophogram; CT useful for other hernias

Differential Diagnosis

Bronchogenic Cyst
- Subcarinal location, will contain air if communicates with GI tract or bronchi

Neurogenic Tumors
- Posterior mediastinal location, no air

Duplication Cyst
- Contain air if ulcerate into GI tract

Sequestration
- Left paraspinal location, systemic arterial supply

Pericardial Cyst
- No air, generally right sided

Diaphragm Hernias

Pathology
<u>General</u>
- Diaphragmatic defects due to congenital failure of fusion of the septum transversum or pleuroperitoneal membranes
- Embryology
  - o Congenital hernias
    - Occurs around 10th week of gestation
    - Hypoplasia lung
    - Lung development determines survival
    - If hernia contains stomach, worse prognosis because gastric herniation occurs earlier in utero
- Epidemiology
  - o Common (sliding hiatal hernia) to rare (paraesophageal)
  - o Sliding: 10% over age 50

<u>Gross Pathologic-Surgical Features</u>
- Sliding hiatal hernia
  - o Atrophy of crura or diaphragmatic muscle
  - o Esophageal hiatus enlarges from increased intra-abdominal pressure
  - o Rotation and mobility of stomach may give rise to gastric volvulus
- Morgagni
  - o Developmental defect between diaphragm muscle and ribs (space of Larrey)
  - o Usually right sided
  - o Rare
- Bochdalek
  - o Developmental or acquired defect pleuroperitoneal hiatus
  - o More common on left
  - o Incidence (<1%)

Clinical Issues
<u>Presentation</u>
- Sliding hernia predisposition: Aging and obesity
- Usually asymptomatic
  - o Reflux: "Heartburn" regurgitation and dysphagia
  - o Occult bleeding
  - o Referred chest pain mimics cardiac disease
  - o Large hernias may cause respiratory compromise
- Gastric volvulus
  - o Triad of Borchardt
    - Pain
    - Unsuccessful vomiting
    - Inability to pass NG tube

<u>Treatment</u>
- Surgery for symptomatic disease
- Antireflux therapy

Selected References
1.   Panicek DM et al: The diaphragm: Anatomic, pathologic, and radiologic considerations. Radiographics 8:385-425, 1988
2.   Goodfellow T et al: Congenital diaphragmatic hernia: The prognostic significance of the site of the stomach. Br J Radiol 60:993-5, 1987
3.   Menuck L et al: Plain film findings of gastric volvulus herniating into the chest. AJR 126:1169-74, 1976

Fibrosing Mediastinitis

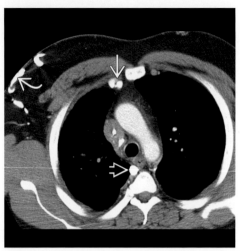

Fibrosing mediastinitis. Right paratracheal mass obstructs SVC. Mass contains central calcification. Note collateral vessels: Right anterior chest wall (curved arrow), right internal mammary vein (arrow), and right superior intercostal vein (open arrow).

Key Facts
- Focal or diffuse mediastinal mass or widening
- Calcification common in focal disease
- Focal disease usually secondary to immune reaction from histoplasmosis
- Diffuse disease usually idiopathic or associated with other autoimmune disease
- Focal disease obstructs SVC, airways, pulmonary veins in that order
- Treatment directed toward stenting airways and vessels

Imaging Findings
General Features
- Best imaging clue: Calcified mediastinal mass with SVC obstruction
Chest Radiograph
- Focal hilar or mediastinal mass or widening
- Focal mass may be calcified
- Lobar collapse with airway obstruction
- SVC syndrome from SVC obstruction
- Pulmonary venous hypertension and interstitial edema from pulmonary vein obstruction
CT Findings
- 80% of focal masses calcified
- Diffuse disease usually not calcified
- Procedure of choice to demonstrate anatomical relationship to surrounding veins and airways
- No contrast enhancement
- Other signs of granulomatous infection
  - Calcified granulomas in lung

Fibrosing Mediastinitis

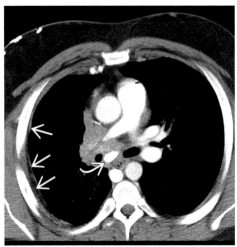

Fibrosing mediastinitis. Superior vena cava obstructed. More inferiorly, mass narrows the right main pulmonary artery. Right hemithorax is slightly smaller. Extrapleural thickening due to enlarged intercostal collaterals (arrows). Subcarinal node is calcified (curved arrow).

<u>Imaging Recommendations</u>
- CT best test to characterize mass and relationship to surrounding structures

Differential Diagnosis
<u>Lymphoma</u>
- Nodular sclerosing Hodgkin's may be difficult to differentiate pathologically
  - o Hodgkin's usually anterior mediastinum
  - o Fibrosing mediastinitis usually hilar, subcarinal and paratracheal
  - o Hodgkin's noncalcified prior to treatment
<u>Bronchogenic Carcinoma</u>
- Bronchogenic carcinoma, no calcification
<u>Bronchogenic Cyst</u>
- Fibrosing mediastinitis not cystic

Pathology
<u>General</u>
- Large biopsy specimen required to exclude lymphoma
- Etiology-pathogenesis
  - o Focal disease thought to arise from abnormal immune response to histoplasmin antigen in susceptible individuals
  - o Diffuse disease unknown cause
<u>Gross Pathologic-Surgical Features</u>
- Focal disease (known as mediastinal granuloma)
  - o Calcified matted nodes containing abundant fibrous tissue
- Diffuse disease
  - o Fibrous tissue replacing mediastinal fat
  - o Must be differentiated from Hodgkin's disease (nodular sclerosing)

Fibrosing Mediastinitis

Erdheim-Chester (Rare, Non-Langerhans Cell Histiocytosis)
- Diffuse encasement aorta and great vessels
- Pleural thickening and perirenal soft tissue encasement
- Sclerotic bone lesions

Microscopic Features
- Benign inflammatory cells, granulomatous response

Clinical Issues
Presentation
- Adults of any age, no sex predilection
- Cough, dyspnea, recurrent pneumonia
- Symptoms related to obstruction, in descending order
  o SVC
  o Airways
  o Pulmonary veins
  o Pulmonary artery
  o Great vessels (protected by high arterial pressure)
- Diffuse disease seen with other autoimmune disorders
  o Retroperitoneal fibrosis
  o Methysergide therapy

Treatment
- Antifungals and steroids ineffective
- Surgery difficult and little benefit
- Palliation
  o Intravascular and airway stents

Prognosis
- Long protracted history, airway compromise or respiratory failure

Selected References
1.   Rossi SE et al: Fibrosing mediastinitis. Radiographics 21:737-57, 2001
2.   Sherrick AD et al: The radiographic findings of fibrosing mediastinitis. Chest 106: 484-9, 1994

Goiter

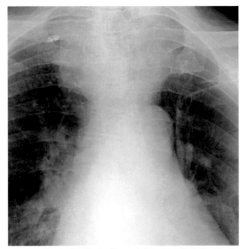

Goiter. Superior mediastinal widening by an inlet mass deviating the trachea to the left.

Key Facts
- Most common cause of tracheal deviation
- Cervical goiters may descend anteriorly (75%) or posteriorly into mediastinum
- Soft tissue high attenuation due to iodine content
- Commonly calcify (coarse, punctate, or rings)
- If hypothyroid may have large pericardial effusion
- Other superior mediastinal masses less likely to deviate trachea
- Usually asymptomatic, symptoms from tracheal or venous compression

Imaging Findings
<u>General Features</u>
- Best imaging clue: Tracheal deviation at level of thoracic inlet
<u>Chest Radiograph</u>
- Tracheal deviation at level of thoracic inlet
- Anterior-superior mediastinal mass or posterior-superior mediastinal mass
- 25% contain calcification
- May have large pericardial effusion if hypothyroid
<u>CT Findings</u>
- Sharply demarcated heterogeneous mass
- Soft tissue attenuation high due to natural iodine
- 75% contain calcification
  - Patterns
    - Coarse
    - Punctate
    - Rings
- Enhances strongly with IV contrast
- Connected to cervical thyroid
- Anterior to trachea (75%)
  - Left side predominant

Goiter

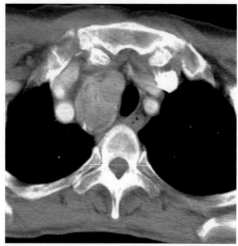

Goiter. Right sided mass contains calcification and several variable sized lower density lesions. Other areas are higher density than soft tissue consistent with iodine containing thyroid tissue.

- Posterior to trachea (25%)
  - Right side predominate

Nuclear Medicine Findings
- I^{123} diagnostic
- Usually not necessary

Imaging Recommendations
- Chest radiography usually sufficient, CT to characterize mass

Differential Diagnosis

Anterior
- Thymoma
  - Less calcification, more caudad in mediastinum, not high attenuation
- Teratoma
  - May have coarse calcification, not of high attenuation, more caudad in mediastinum
- Lymphoma
  - Not calcified prior to treatment, usually multiple nodes

Posterior
- Bronchogenic cyst
  - May be of high attenuation due to milk of calcium, non-enhancing
- Leiomyosarcoma esophagus
  - Not of high attenuation, no calcification
- Bronchogenic carcinoma
  - No calcification, ill-defined margins

Pathology

General
- Thyroid hyperplasia with colloid distended follicles
- Etiology-pathogenesis

Goiter

- o Dietary absence of iodine leads to insufficient production of thyroid hormone
- o Excess thyroid-stimulating hormone (TSH)
- o Uniform enlargement initially eventually leads to differential growth

Gross Pathologic-Surgical Features
- Enlarged thyroid, heterogeneous, cystic degeneration, hemorrhage, calcification

Microscopic Features
- Irregularly enlarged follicles with flattened epithelium and abundant colloid

Clinical Issues

Presentation
- Mostly women
- Common, 25% cervical goiters descend into thorax
- Usually asymptomatic and euthyroid
- Tracheal compression
  - o Dyspnea
  - o Wheezing
  - o Stridor
- Pemberton's sign
  - o Neck vein distention with upper extremity elevation

Treatment
- Surgery for symptomatic disease
- Iodine replacement
- Thyroid replacement for hypothyroidism

Selected References
1. Buckley JA et al: Intrathoracic mediastinal thyroid goiter: Imaging manifestations. AJR 173:471-5, 1999
2. Bashist B et al: Computed tomography of intrathoracic goiters. AJR 140:455-60, 1983

Pneumomediastinum

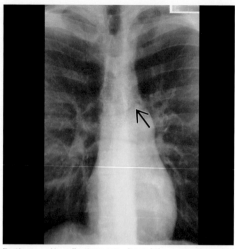

Pneumomediastinum. Air collections may be subtle on the frontal view (arrow). History of asthma.

Key Facts
- Intrathoracic (Valsalva) and extrathoracic (sinus, dental, duodenal) causes
- Trauma: Blunt chest trauma, bronchial tear, esophageal tear
- Best seen lateral view
- Differentiate from other air: Does not shift with decubitus films
- Hamman's sign (precordial crunching)
- May be fatal in neonates: Tension pneumomediastinum

Imaging Findings
General Features
- Best imaging clue: Air outlining heart and mediastinal vessels on lateral radiograph

Chest Radiograph
- Signs
  - Thymic sail
  - Ring around the artery
  - Tubular artery sign
  - Double bronchial wall
  - Continuous diaphragm
  - Extrapleural sign
  - Naclerio's V sign
    - Costovertebral air adjacent to hemidiaphragm and spine
  - Subcutaneous emphysema
- Best seen lateral view

CT Findings
- More sensitive, identical to chest radiograph

Imaging Recommendations
- Chest radiograph useful for detection, CT occasionally useful

Pneumomediastinum

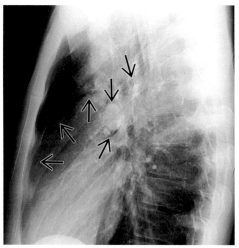

Pneumomediastinum is often easier to detect on the lateral film. Air outlines (arrows) the heart and great vessels. Air may also surround bronchi.

Differential Diagnosis

Pneumothorax
- Air will shift with position, visceral pleural line smooth, extrapleural line not smooth and usually thicker
- Usually unilateral, extrapleural sign often bilateral

Pneumopericardium
- Less common in adults, air confined to pericardium

Mach Band
- Due to retinal inhibition, obscuring one edge with finger or hand will make mach band disappear
- Convex soft-tissue density into concave lung density = black Mach band, example heart border
- Convex lung density into concave soft tissue density = white Mach band, example paraesophageal stripe

Pathology

General
- Not a pathologic diagnosis
- Etiology-pathogenesis
  - Macklin effect
    - Alveolar rupture leads to
    - Pulmonary interstitial emphysema: PIE in infants; rarely seen in adults leads to pneumomediastinum
  - Causes
    - Sustained Valsalva: Asthma, cough, weight lifting, straining, marijuana use
    - Blunt chest trauma
    - Bronchial fracture: consider if progressively worsens
    - Esophageal tear: Naclerio's V sign
    - Spontaneous
    - Sinus fracture

Pneumomediastinum

- Dental extraction
- Positive pressure ventilation
- Duodenal ulcer: Sigmoid diverticulitis

Clinical Issues

Presentation
- Serious in neonates
  - Vascular collapse due to venous obstruction
    - Adults decompress into neck or retroperitoneum
  - PIE: Air block
    - Interstitial vascular compression
- Chest pain
- Dyspnea
- Hamman's sign
  - Precordial "crunch" at auscultation
    - Like the noise of peas rattling on taut canvas
- May lead to pneumothorax, pneumoperitoneum, retroperitoneal air

Treatment
- None, observe for pneumothorax
- Treat underlying cause

Prognosis
- Benign except in neonates
- Morbidity and mortality related to etiology

Selected References
1. Zylak et al: Pneumomediastinum revisited. Radiographics 20:1043-57, 2000
2. Bejvan SM et al: Pneumomediastinum: Old signs and new signs. AJR 166:1041-8, 1996
3. Cyrlak D et al: Pneumomediastinum: A diagnostic problem. Crit Rev Diagn Imaging 23:75-117, 1984

Esophageal Disease

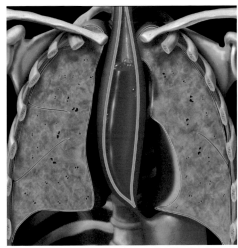

Achalasia. Markedly dilated esophagus with an air fluid level at the upper esophagus and beaking at the esophagogastric junction. Typically there is no air fluid level seen in the stomach on upright chest radiographs.

Key Facts
- Thickening posterior tracheal stripe clue to underlying esophageal disease
- Diffuse mediastinal widening with air-fluid level suggests achalasia
- Esophageal masses rarely large enough for detection chest radiograph
- Esophogram key to evaluate motility, reflux, and aspiration

Imaging Findings
General Features
- Best imaging clue: Thickening posterior tracheal stripe
Chest Radiograph
- Thickening posterior tracheal stripe (normally < 4.5 mm thickness)
  - Lymphatics run longitudinally so that lower esophageal pathology from inflammation or neoplasia will thicken posterior tracheal stripe
- Achalasia
  - Diffuse mediastinal widening, air-fluid level upper mediastinum posterior to trachea
  - Absence gastric air bubble
- Varices
  - Visible in up to 30% of patients with portal hypertension
  - Small liver, enlarged spleen
  - Obliteration of edge of descending aorta
- Sclerotherapy for varices
  - Pleural effusion 30%, mediastinal widening 35%
  - Left basilar opacities 5%, pneumomediastinum < 1%
- Perforation, Boerhaave's
  - Pneumomediastinum left costovertebral angle (V-sign of Naclerio)
  - Mediastinal widening, pneumothorax or hydropneumothorax
  - Pleural effusion
    - Tear mid-esophagus mainly right hemithorax
    - Tear lower esophagus mainly left hemithorax

Esophageal Disease

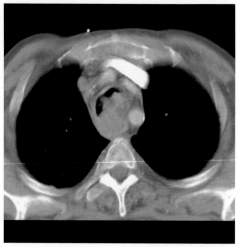

Large esophageal carcinoma at the level of the left subclavian artery invading the trachea.

- Esophageal mass
  - Carcinoma or leiomyomas are rarely of sufficient size to be evident
  - Carcinoma may obstruct esophagus causing dilatation but not to the degree seen in achalasia
  - Diverticula may have air-fluid level and have tendency to extend into right hemithorax

<u>CT Findings</u>
- Useful to evaluate esophageal masses and surrounding extension

<u>Esophogram Findings</u>
- Procedure of choice to evaluate esophageal motility, reflux, and aspiration
- Possible perforation should be evaluated with barium or nonionic contrast, gastrografin should be avoided because of the risks of aspiration
- Achalasia: Absence primary peristalsis, smooth tapering distal esophagus "beak-like" dilated esophagus has sigmoid configuration

Differential Diagnosis
<u>Neurogenic Tumors</u>
- Short lesion, dilated esophagus is long lesion, no air in neurogenic tumors

<u>Aortic Dissection or Aneurysms</u>
- Long lesion, no air, rim calcification

<u>Bronchogenic Cysts</u>
- May contain air if communicate with GI tract or bronchus, subcarinal location

Pathology
<u>Achalasia</u>
- Etiology unknown
- Pathophysiology: Myenteric plexus neuropathy with incomplete relaxation lower esophageal sphincter
- Esophagitis, secondary to stasis of esophageal contents

Esophageal Disease

- Secondary causes: Esophageal carcinoma, metastases, lymphoma, Chagas disease, vagotomy

Varices
- Dilatation paraesophageal veins from portal hypertension

Boerhaave Perforation
- Left posterolateral wall of esophagus superior to esophagogastric junction

Diverticula
- Proximal: Zenker's pulsion through cricoesophageal membrane
- Mid: Traction diverticula from adjacent granulomatous lymph nodes
- Lower: Epiphrenic pulsion

Esophageal Carcinoma
- 95% squamous cell carcinoma
- 5% adenocarcinomas

Clinical Issues

General
- Dysphagia, chest pain, hemoptysis

Achalasia
- Middle age, M=F
- Dysphagia (90%)
- Recurrent pneumonias

Varices
- Chronic liver disease causing portal hypertension
- Bleeding controlled with sclerotherapy
- Sclerotherapy complications include perforation, aspiration, and ARDS from embolized sclerotherapy agents

Perforation
- Causes
  o Boerhaave follows vomiting or blunt chest trauma
  o Instrumentation, endoscopy, following esophageal dilatation for achalasia or balloon tamponade for variceal bleeding
- Subcutaneous crepitus neck

Esophageal Carcinoma
- Usually advanced disease at diagnosis

Diverticula
- Pulsion diverticula arise as a complication of motility disorder
- Traction diverticula a result of adjacent inflammatory disease, usually healed lymph nodes from histoplasmosis

Treatment
- Achalasia: Pneumatic dilatation risk of perforation
- Perforation: Drainage, antibiotics, surgical closure
- Carcinoma: Radiation, total esophagectomy, usually from a right thoracotomy approach (Ivor-Lewis)

Prognosis
- Variable, diverticula generally benign, carcinoma prognosis poor
- Perforation: Delayed diagnosis has high morbidity and mortality

Selected References
1. Stark P et al: Manifestations of esophageal disease on plain chest radiographs. AJR 155:729-34, 1990
2. Gedgaudas-McClees RK et al: Thoracic findings in gastrointestinal pathology. Radiol Clin North Am 22:563-89, 1984

Nerve Sheath Tumors

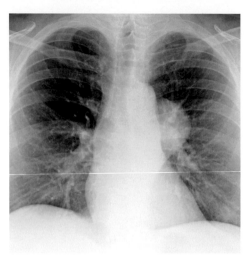

Sharply marginated mass in the posterior mediastinum (lateral chest radiograph not shown). Differential would include aneurysm, bronchogenic cyst, and neurogenic tumors. Chest otherwise normal.

Key Facts
- Most common cause of posterior mediastinal mass
- Centered on neural foramen
- Round shape and horizontal axis
- Decreased attenuation at CT due to lipid or cystic degeneration
- Neurofibromas have target appearance at MRI and enhance with gadolinium
- Neurofibromas associated with von Recklinghausen disease

Imaging Findings
General Features
- Best imaging clue: Round posterior mediastinal mass with widened neural foramen
Chest Radiograph
- Shape: Round, sharply marginated
- Length: Extends 1-2 rib interspaces
- Long axis: Horizontal, follows intercostal nerves
  - Dumbbell extension into spinal canal (10%)
  - Centered at neural foramen, widens foramen
- Scoliosis upper thoracic spine
CT Findings
- Decreased attenuation due to lipid, cystic degeneration
- Variable enhancement (homogeneous, heterogeneous) with IV contrast
MRI Findings
- Useful to evaluate intraspinal extension
- Neurofibroma
  - Central position within nerve
  - Target appearance with high peripheral signal on T2WI
  - Enhance with gadolinium
- Generally low signal T1 and high signal T2

Nerve Sheath Tumors

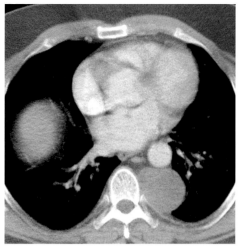

CT with IV contrast. Sharply marginated low-density mass in the posterior mediastinum. Adjacent vertebral body and ribs normal. CT demonstrates that this lesion is not vascular. Surgically removed, diagnosis: Neurofibroma.

<u>Malignant Degeneration (Malignant Tumor of Nerve Sheath Origin)</u>
- Neither CT nor MRI useful to distinguish malignant vs benign tumors
  - Sudden increase in size suspicious for malignancy
  - Indistinct margins more common with malignancy

Differential Diagnosis
<u>Sympathetic Ganglion Tumor</u>
- Oval shape and vertical axis
- Extends over 3-5 interspaces
- More often calcified
<u>Paraganglioma</u>
- Paraganglioma strongly enhance with contrast
<u>Esophageal Duplication Cyst</u>
- Esophageal duplication cyst more anterior, lower attenuation, fluid characteristics at MRI

Pathology
<u>General</u>
- 90% of all posterior mediastinal masses neurogenic origin
  - 40% of these nerve sheath tumors
  - 3:1 schwannomas to neurofibromas
- Genetics
  - 30% associated with von Recklinghausen disease (Neurofibromatosis 1) chromosome 17 deletion
  - Neurofibromatosis–2, chromosome 22q deletion
- Epidemiology
  - Age 30-40s
  - M=F
  - Neurofibromas 90% solitary, rarely undergo malignant degeneration

Nerve Sheath Tumors

- o Neurofibromatosis malignant degeneration 4%
- o Schwannomas rarely undergo malignant degeneration
- o Neurofibromatosis-1: Prevalence 1 in 3,000
  - ▪ Other tumors: Pheochromocytoma, CML
- o Neurofibromatosis-2: Prevalence 1 in 1,000,000

Gross Pathologic-Surgical Findings
- • Schwannomas
  - o Encapsulated nerve sheath tumors eccentrically compress nerve
  - o Often undergo cystic degeneration and hemorrhage
- • Neurofibroma
  - o Nonencapsulated disorganized proliferation of all nerve elements, centrally positioned in nerve

Microscopic Findings
- • Neurofibroma: Myelinated and unmyelinated axons, collagen, reticulin
- • Schwannoma: Antoni A (highly cellular) or B (loose myxoid)

Clinical Issues

Presentation
- • Usually asymptomatic
- • Symptoms variable related to mass effect or nerve entrapment

Treatment
- • Surgical removal for symptomatic or malignant lesions
- • Radiation not indicated, may induce malignant degeneration

Prognosis
- • 5-year survival malignant lesions 35%

Selected References
1. Strollo DC et al: Primary mediastinal tumors: Part II. Tumors of the middle and posterior mediastinum. Chest 112:1344-57, 1997
2. Reed JC et al: Neural tumors of the thorax: Subject review from the AFIP. Radiology 126:9-17, 1978

Sympathetic Ganglion Tumors

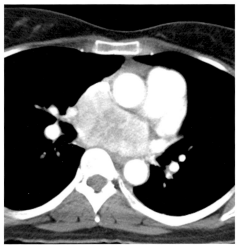

Paraganglioma. CT with contrast. Large enhancing subcarinal mass. Differential includes carcinoid, parathyroid tumors, and granulomatous lymph nodes.

Key Facts
- Common posterior mediastinal mass
- Oval shape and vertical axis spanning 3 to 5 vertebra
- Malignant tumors usually calcified
- Age related: Neuroblastoma < 3, ganglioneuroblastoma 3-10, ganglioneuroma > 10
- Neuroblastoma associated with paraneoplastic syndromes
- Paraganglioma arise from parasympathetic ganglia (may produce catecholamines)

Imaging Findings
<u>General Features</u>
- Best imaging clue: Elongated vertical posterior mediastinal mass

<u>Chest Radiograph</u>
- Shape: Oval sharply marginated
- Length: Extend 3-5 rib interspaces
- Long axis: Vertical, follows sympathetic chain
  - Erodes ribs and vertebral bodies
  - Spreads ribs
- Calcification: 80% in neuroblastoma
  - Malignant tumors more likely to have calcification than benign tumors

<u>CT Findings</u>
- Heterogeneous due to hemorrhage, cystic degeneration and necrosis
- More malignant the tumor the more likely the degree of heterogeneity
- Variable enhancement (homogeneous, heterogeneous) with IV contrast
- Paragangliomas strongly and uniformly enhance with contrast
  - Other common locations: Intrapericardial (difficult to separate from ventricular contrast) and aortic arch-great vessels

<u>MRI Findings</u>
- Useful to evaluate intraspinal extension
- Ganglioneuroma

Sympathetic Ganglion Tumors

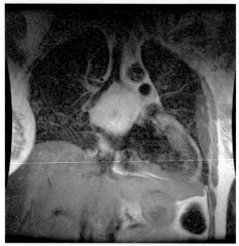

Paraganglioma. Coronal T1 weighted sequence with gadolinium. Tumor diffusely enhances with contrast. Left atrium is compressed and carina is splayed.

- o Whorled appearance T1WI
- o Enhance with gadolinium
- Generally low signal T1 and high T2
- Paraganglioma strongly enhance with gadolinium

Imaging Recommendations
- CT to characterize mass, MRI useful for intraspinal extension

Differential Diagnosis

Nerve Sheath Tumor
- Neurofibromas may be multiple
- Nerve sheath tumors in older individuals
- Horizontal axis, round, centered on neural foramen

Esophageal Duplication Cyst
- Esophageal duplication cyst more anterior, lower attenuation, fluid characteristics at MRI or CT

Pathology

General
- Spectrum from malignancy to benign ganglion cells
- Epidemiology
  - o 90% of all posterior mediastinal masses neurogenic origin
  - o 65% of these sympathetic ganglion tumors
  - o Paraganglioma extremely rare (<0.5% mediastinal tumors)

Gross Pathologic-Surgical Features
- Neuroblastoma
  - o Nonencapsulated
  - o Inhomogeneous: hemorrhage, necrosis, cystic degeneration
- Ganglioneuroblastoma
  - o More homogeneous in between neuroblastoma and ganglioneuroma
- Ganglioneuroma
  - o Encapsulated

- o Homogeneous soft tissue density
- Paraganglioma
  - o Arises from neural crest, often highly vascular
  - o Produce catecholamines (then are called pheochromocytoma)

Microscopic Features
- Neuroblastoma: Small round cells arranged in sheets
- Ganglioneuroma: Clustered mature ganglion cells
- Ganglioneuroblastoma: Admixture of neuroblastoma and ganglioneuroma
- Paraganglioma: Vascular spaces mixed with APUD cells

Staging: Sympathetic Ganglion Tumors
- Stage I: Ipsilateral noninvasive
- Stage II: Ipsilateral locally invasive
- Stage III: Extension across midline and/or regional lymph nodes
- Stage IV: Widespread metastases (liver, skin, bone)

Clinical Issues

Presentation
- Usually asymptomatic
- Neuroblastoma
  - o Children < 3
  - o Most common extra-adrenal location
- Ganglioneuroblastoma
  - o Children < 10
- Ganglioneuroma
  - o Adolescents and young adults
- Neuroblastoma may have paraneoplastic syndrome
  - o VIP induced watery diarrhea
  - o Achlorhydria
  - o Hypokalemia
  - o Opsomyoclonus
    - ▪ Cerebellar ataxia
    - ▪ Nystagmus
    - ▪ Myoclonus
- Paraganglioma
  - o Adults, blushing, headaches with catecholamine secretion

Natural History
- Neuroblastoma may mature to a ganglioneuroblastoma, then ganglioneuroma

Treatment
- Surgical resection
- Adjuvant chemotherapy and radiation therapy for advanced disease

Selected References
1.   Strollo DC et al: Primary mediastinal tumors: Part II. Tumors of the middle and posterior mediastinum. Chest 112:1344-57, 1997
2.   Reed JC et al: Neural tumors of the thorax: Subject review from the AFIP. Radiology 126:9-17, 1978

PocketRadiologist™
Chest
Top 100 Diagnoses

CARCINOMA

Lung Cancer Staging

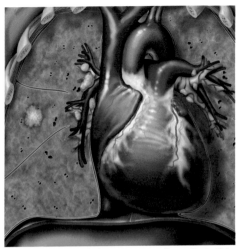

Noncalcified irregular nodule in right lung measures < 3 cm. The ipsilateral right hilar nodes are enlarged with metastatic tumor. Stage IIa non-small cell lung carcinoma.

Key Facts
- Staging determines anatomic extent, treatment and prognosis
- CT impact
  - Decrease number of open-close thoracotomies
  - Decrease number resections in patients with occult metastases
  - Improves surgical and radiation therapy planning
- Up to 1/3 of patients surgically resected probably have metastases
- CT nodal staging: 20% false positives and 20% false negatives
- Prevalence of metastases in normal-sized lymph nodes: 15%

Imaging Findings
General Features
- Best imaging clue: Mediastinal nodes greater than 4 cm metastatic
CT Findings
- Abnormal nodes > 1 cm short axis diameter
  - Normal nodes vary in size by mediastinal region
    - Subcarinal nodes may be up to 12 mm in short axis diameter
- Accuracy of CT nodal staging
  - 20% false positives, 20% false negatives
  - Frequency of nodal metastases (20 to 50%)
  - Frequency of metastases nodes over 3 cm (66%)
  - Frequency of metastases nodes over 4 cm (100%)
  - Frequency of metastases normal-sized nodes (15%)
- Accuracy of CT T_4
  - Simple contact chest wall or mediastinum
    - 50% accuracy (coin toss)
    - Patients may be curable, T_4 should be surgically confirmed
- Value of asymptomatic extrathoracic staging for M_1
  - Head CT: 3% frequency metastases
  - Adrenal CT: 5% frequency metastases

Lung Cancer Staging

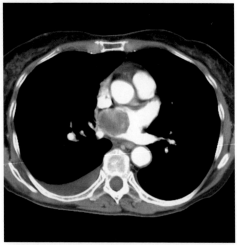

Tumor has grown down the right superior pulmonary vein into the left atrium. Small right pleural effusion. T_4 tumor (invasion of heart) and is at minimum Stage IIIb, which is unresectable.

- o Bone scan: 9% frequency metastases
- o Liver imaging: 2% frequency metastases
- Adrenal evaluation
  - o 5% normal population have incidental adrenal mass
  - o Nonenhanced CT
    - Adenomas < 10 HU (due to lipid)
    - ROI should be 1/3 to 1/2 size of lesion
    - 98% specific, 70% sensitive for adenomas
  - o Enhanced CT
  - o % Enhancement washout = (Enhanced $CT_{attenuation}$ − Delayed $CT_{attenuation}$)/ (Enhanced $CT_{attenuation}$ − Unenhanced $CT_{attenuation}$) × 100
    - Adenomas > 60% washout
    - Sensitivity 86%, specificity 92%
  - o % Relative washout = (Enhanced $CT_{attenuation}$ − Delayed $CT_{attenuation}$)/ Enhanced $CT_{attenuation}$ × 100
    - Adenomas > 40% washout
    - Sensitivity 82%, specificity 92%

MRI Findings
- Accuracy similar to CT
- Slightly superior to CT for chest wall invasion
- Coronal plane advantageous for superior sulcus tumors

Differential Diagnosis
- None

Pathology
General
- Non-small cell carcinoma, in order of frequency
  - o Adenocarcinoma > squamous cell carcinoma > large cell carcinoma
- Prevalence of metastases in normal-sized nodes: 15%

Lung Cancer Staging

- Adenocarcinoma 2x as likely as squamous cell carcinoma to metastasize to nodes or brain

Staging TNM Non-Small Cell Carcinoma
- T_1: SPN < 3 cm diameter
- T_2
  - Mass > 3 cm
  - Any tumor invading visceral pleura
  - Any tumor causing endobronchial atelectasis (less than whole lung)
    - Must be 2 cm distal to carina
- T_3
  - Any tumor extending into chest wall, diaphragm, mediastinal fat, or pericardium
  - Whole lung atelectasis
  - < 2 cm from carina
- T_4
  - Any tumor invading heart, great vessels, trachea, esophagus, vertebral body, carina
  - Malignant pleural effusion
- N_0: No nodes
- N_1: Ipsilateral hilar nodes, includes subcarinal nodes
- N_2: Ipsilateral mediastinal nodes
- N_3: Contralateral mediastinal, ipsilateral scalene, or supraclavicular nodes
- Small cell carcinoma
  - Staging: Limited or Extensive
    - Limited: To thorax (amenable to radiation therapy port)
    - Extensive: Widespread disease

Survival
- Stage Ia (T_1N_0) 65% 5- year survival
- Stage Ib (T_2N_0) 40% 5- year survival
- Stage IIa (T_1N_1) 35% 5- year survival
- Stage IIb (T_2N_1, T_3N_0) 25% 5- year survival
- Stage IIIa ($T_{1-3}N_2$, T_3N_1) 10% 5- year survival
- Stage IIIb ($T_{1-4}N_3$, T_4N_{0-3}) 5% 5- year survival
- Stage IV (M_1) 1% 5- year survival

Clinical Issues
Presentation
- Symptoms usually not evident until advanced disease
- Unresectable: T_4, N_3, M_1 ($\geq$ Stage IIIb)
- Patient should be given the benefit of proof, denying surgery currently precludes chance of cure
- Without screening, most patients present with symptoms and advanced Stage III disease (borderline resectable)

Treatment
- Surgery < Stage IIIb
- Unresectable disease, palliative radiation therapy and chemotherapy

Selected References
1. Ellis SM et al: Computed tomography screening for lung cancer: Back to basics. Clin Radiol 56:691-9, 2001
2. Strauss GM: Randomized population trials and screening for lung cancer: Breaking the cure barrier. Cancer 89: 2399-421, 2000
3. Henschke CI et al: Early Lung Cancer Action Project: Overall design and findings from baseline screening. Lancet 354:99-105, 1999

Radiation Therapy

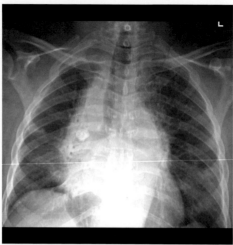

Diffuse mediastinal widening. Mediastinal borders are straight with ill-defined margins, which appear to extend into the lung. History of radiation therapy for Hodgkins disease. Radiation fibrosis paramediastinal lung conforming to mantle port. Differential would include recurrrent adenopathy.

Key Facts
- Radiation pneumonitis near constant over 40 Gy
- Pathology: Nonspecific diffuse alveolar damage
- Radiologic course 1 to 12 months following completion of therapy
- Radiation effect potentiated by chemotherapy
- Symptoms alleviated by steroids

Imaging Findings
General Features
- Best imaging clue: Nonanatomic consolidation and volume loss confined to port
Chest Radiograph
- Chronologic sequence (Rule of 4's)
  - 4 weeks to deliver therapy of 40 Gy
  - 4 weeks after end of therapy
    - Earliest radiographic manifestation: Indistinct vessel margins in radiated lung
  - 4 months after end of therapy
    - Peak radiation pneumonitis: Focal consolidation; may not involve entire volume irradiated lung
  - 12 (4x3) months after end of therapy
    - Gradual clearing consolidated lung
    - Progressive volume loss in radiated lung
    - Sharp nonanatomic boundaries conforming to portal
    - Stabilization after 12 to 18 months
    - Any increase in density or growth: Suspect metastatic disease
  - Sequence accelerated 1 week for each extra 10 Gy of therapy
- Treated Hodgkin's disease
  - May develop thymic cysts
  - Abnormal nodes may calcify after therapy

Radiation Therapy

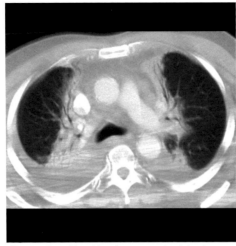

CT radiation fibrosis. Consolidated lung has non-anatomic borders corresponding to the port from Mantle therapy. Small bilateral pleural effusions. No adenopathy.

- o Eggshell or mulberry type calcification
- Bone
  - o Cortical thickening after 12 months
  - o Fractures 2-3 years post therapy
  - o Aseptic necrosis
  - o Osteochondromas (up to 10% in children)
  - o Osteosarcomas latent period averages 15 years

CT Findings
- More sensitive than chest radiography for radiation changes
  - o Same as radiography
  - o May see patchy opacities that extend beyond the port (BOOP)
  - o Pleural and pericardial effusions
  - o Bronchiectasis within the port
  - o Hyper lucent oligemic lung beyond the port
  - o Volume loss in affected lung, architectural distortion
- Modality of choice to detect recurrent disease

Imaging Recommendations
- Chest radiographs for detection and course, CT useful if question of recurrent disease

Differential Diagnosis

Infection
- Radiation effect generally limited to port, knowledge of port geometry essential

Drug-Induced Toxicity
- Radiation effect generally limited to port, knowledge of port geometry essential

Recurrent or Metastatic Neoplasm
- Any contour or density change after 12 months suggestive of recurrence
- Cicatricial fibrosis contains air bronchograms
  - o Loss of air bronchograms suggests recurrence

Radiation Therapy

Pathology

General
- Nonspecific, diffuse, alveolar damage generally limited to radiation port
- Natural history
  - Phases
  - Acute exudative
    - Alveolar wall thickening
    - Proteinaceous edema
    - Mononuclear cell infiltrate
    - Proliferation type II pneumocytes
    - Hyaline membrane formation
  - Organizing proliferative
    - Incorporation hyaline membranes
    - Collagen deposition
    - Regeneration alveolar epithelium
  - Chronic fibrosis
    - Cicatricial atelectasis
    - Honeycombing
- Etiology-pathogenesis
  - Dose dependent
    - Rare < 20 Gy
    - Universal > 40 Gy
    - Considerable individual variation
    - Other factors: Total dose, duration, fractionation schedule, volume irradiated, potentiated with chemotherapy

Microscopic Features
- Nonspecific, diffuse alveolar disease (DAD) inflammatory cells acutely, end-stage fibrosis when healed

Clinical Issues

Presentation
- Symptoms dependent on severity and volume of irradiated lung
- Symptoms nonspecific: Dyspnea, nonproductive cough, fever

Treatment
- Short term steroids for symptomatic cases

Prognosis
- Related to underlying malignancy

Selected References
1. Logan PM: Thoracic manifestations of external beam radiotherapy. AJR 171:569-577, 1998
2. Libshitz HI et al: Complications of radiation therapy: The thorax. Semin Roentgenol 9:41-9, 1974

Missed Lung Cancer & Screening

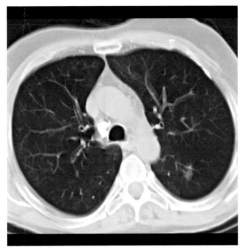

Screening CT. 7 mm indeterminate nodule left lower lobe. The probability of detecting such a nodule from a chest radiograph is < 50%.

Key Facts
- Missed lung cancer 2nd most common malpractice litigation (breast cancer #1)
- Comparison with prior films most important method to reduce errors
- Sensitivity of chest radiography for Stage I lung cancer 15%
- Endpoint of screening studies is reduction in mortality, not increase in 5-year survival
- Screening with sputum cytology or chest radiography has not been shown to reduce mortality
- Lung cancer screening with CT shows promise

Imaging Findings
<u>General Features</u>
- Best imaging clue: Most missed cancers in the upper lobes
<u>Chest Radiograph</u>
- Most common location of lung cancer is upper lobes
- Most common location missed lung cancer is upper lobes
- Observer has 50% chance to detect a nodule 1 cm in diameter
  - Factors affecting detection
    - Film quality, lesion size, lesion conspicuity, overlap of vessels and chest wall structures, ill-defined edges
  - Satisfaction of search
- Hierarchy of errors
  - 45% poor decision making: Lesion seen but dismissed as insignificant
  - 35% recognition error: Fixated on lesion but not brought to level of consciousness of observer
  - 20% scanning error: Observer never focused on abnormality
<u>Screening</u>
- 5 year survival lung cancer 15%, hasn't changed in 40 years
- Those presenting with symptoms (the majority) have advanced disease

Missed Lung Cancer & Screening

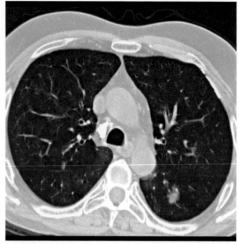

Short term 3 month follow-up. The nodule has grown and was surgically resected. Stage I non-small cell carcinoma. The role of CT for screening is considered investigational and may not decrease mortality.

- Screening with sputum cytology or chest radiography has not reduced mortality
  - Previous results of randomized trials controversial
- Sensitivity of chest radiography to detect Stage I lung cancer 15%
- Endpoint of screening is reduction of mortality, not increase 5-year survival; Survival subject to bias in nonrandomized studies

Lead Time Bias
- Example: 2 identical smokers, one screened the other not, both develop lung cancer at the same time
- Screened individual has lung cancer diagnosed, he dies 6 years later of metastases, survival is 6 years
- Nonscreened individual is discovered to have lung cancer (symptomatic) 5 years after the screened individual and dies 1 year later, survival 1 year
- The difference in survival is lead time, mortality is the same

Overdiagnosis Bias
- False-positive pathology for cancer
  - "Resected" lung cancer long survival
- Clinically unimportant tumors (length time bias)
  - Growth so slow or indolent as not to affect the health of the individual
    - Documented for prostate and thyroid carcinoma
    - Autopsy evidence for occult lung cancer (1%)
    - However, in NCI lung cancer detection program: 45 unresected Stage I lung cancer only 2 survived 5 years (4.4%)

NCI Lung Cancer Detection Programs
- Johns Hopkins (JH), Memorial Sloan Kettering (MSK), Mayo Clinic (MC)
- 6 year screen
- JH and MSK both control and interventional groups had chest radiograph, only variable was sputum cytology
- MC, interventional group has chest radiograph every 4 months, control group advised to have chest radiograph

Missed Lung Cancer & Screening

- Approximately 50% of the control group followed advice had chest radiography, contaminating the effect of chest x-ray screening
- In none was mortality decreased in the interventional group (actually mortality increased but not statistically significant)

CT Screening
- Lung cancer screening with low dose CT
  - Low dose
    - 40 mA multislice, 80 mA single slice
    - Dose 1/10 that of conventional CT
- In comparison to chest radiography
  - Average size primary tumor size decreased by 50%
  - Proportion of Stage I tumors nearly doubled
  - 4x as many tumors detected compared to chest radiography
- Early Lung Cancer Action Project (ELCAP)
  - 1000 smokers older than 60
  - 85% (23/27) Stage I lung cancers
  - 2nd incidence scan 70% (5/7) Stage I lung cancer
  - Nonrandomized, results may be biased
  - 13% (4/30) of cancers missed on prior CT
    - Emphasizes that false negatives possible
  - Mayo Clinic nonrandomized study
    - 50% screened have indeterminate nodules
    - False positives expensive to follow
    - Some undergo unnecessary surgery

Differential Diagnosis
General
- Solitary pulmonary nodule (SPN) 90% due to granuloma, bronchogenic carcinoma, metastasis, hamartoma, carcinoid
- False positives usually due to granuloma, distribution of fungi that cause granulomas varies considerably worldwide

Pathology
General
- Average doubling time of bronchogenic carcinoma 100 days (40–400 days)

Clinical Issues
General
- Missed lung cancer significant medical-legal problem
- Lung cancer screening with CT undergoing randomized trial

Selected References
1. Ellis SM et al: Computed tomography screening for lung cancer: Back to basics. Clin Radiol 56:691-9, 2001
2. Strauss GM: Randomized population trials and screening for lung cancer: Breaking the cure barrier Cancer 89:2399-421, 2000
3. Henschke CI et al: Early Lung Cancer Action Project: Overall design and findings from baseline screening. Lancet 354:99-105, 1999

PocketRadiologist™
Chest
Top 100 Diagnoses

NODULE(S)

Solitary Pulmonary Nodule (SPN)

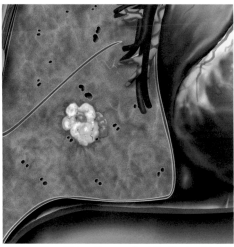

Hamartoma. CT detection of fat and "popcorn" calcification in a lobulated soft tissue nodule < 2.5 cm in diameter suggests diagnosis. Slow growing and usually detected in 4th or 5th decade of life.

Key Facts
- Common radiographic problem – goal is to separate benign from malignant
- Up to 40% of SPNs may be curable lung cancer
- 90% represent (in order) granuloma, bronchogenic carcinoma, hamartoma, solitary metastasis, carcinoid
- Benign calcification pitfalls – osteogenic carcinoma, carcinoid tumor
- Contrast enhancement of SPN sensitive but poor specificity
- PET pitfalls: Small (< 7 mm diameter), carcinoid, bronchioloalveolar cell carcinoma
- Hamartoma more likely to contain fat than calcium

Imaging Findings
General Features
- Best imaging clue: 50% chance to detect 7 mm non-calcified nodule
Chest Radiograph
- Definition: Isolated rounded pulmonary density < 3 cm in diameter
- Often missed
  - Up to 90% visible in retrospect in screening lung cancer studies
    - Conspicuity (overlapping structures)
    - Faulty search pattern
  - Calcification benign patterns
    - Central nidus, laminated, diffuse, "popcorn"
  - Calcification pitfalls
    - 1/3 carcinoids calcified, central lesions may have central nidus
    - Osteogenic sarcoma metastasis may be diffusely calcified
  - Growth
    - Benign: None or doubling time > 2 years
    - Typical malignancy 100 day doubling time
    - Old films **CRITICAL**

Solitary Pulmonary Nodule (SPN)

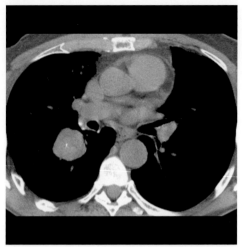

Hamartoma. Large lobulated SPN with tiny nidus of calcification. Hamartomas are twice as likely to contain fat as calcium. Differential would include granuloma, bronchogenic carcinoma and carcinoid. The latter often develops adjacent to lobar and segmental bronchus and may contain a nidus of calcification.

- o Benign characteristics (malignant characteristics in parenthesis)
  - Sharp edge (ill-defined)
  - Round shape (spiculated)
  - Lower lobe location (upper lobe)
  - Satellite lesions (solitary)
- Hamartoma
  - o Popcorn calcification
    - Carney's triad: 1. multiple chondromas, 2. gastric leiomyoma (sarcoma), 3. extra-adrenal paraganglioma

CT Findings
- Utility
  - o True nodule or artifact
  - o Single or multiple
  - o Stage if lung cancer
- 10x more sensitive technique to detect calcification
  - o > 200 HU considered calcified
- Contrast enhancement
  - o Densitometry following IV contrast bolus
  - o Related to angiogenesis and blood flow
  - o 15 HU threshold, benign < 15, malignant > 20
    - Sensitivity 98% specificity 60%
- Fat
  - o Benign finding, found in hamartomas and lipoma
- Hamartoma
  - o 1/3 contain fat (1/4 contain calcium)
- Carcinoid
  - o Central lesion adjacent to lobar or segmental bronchi may have central calcified nidus
  - o May have striking contrast enhancement

Solitary Pulmonary Nodule (SPN)

PET Findings
- Measure glucose metabolism
- False negatives: Carcinoid, bronchioloalveolar cell carcinoma, or tumors < 7 mm in size
- Sensitivity: 95% specificity 90%

Differential Diagnosis
Mimics
- 1st costochondral junction
  - Inferior aspect 1st rib, more common right (right-handed)
- Pulmonary vein confluence
  - Upper aspect right heart border
- Nipple shadow
  - Bilateral, outer edge sharp, inner edge indistinct

Pathologic Features
General
- Etiology-pathogenesis
  - Granulomas calcify earlier in young individuals
- Epidemiology
  - Age increases probability of malignancy
  - Prevalence of granulomas depends on indigenous fungi
  - Cigarette consumption, direct dose (tar) relationship with lung cancer
  - Carcinoma: adenocarcinoma most common type to present as SPN
Gross Pathologic Features
- SPN characteristics useful in separating benign and malignant
Microscopic Features
- Depends on pathology

Clinical Issues
Presentation
- Asymptomatic, usually incidental finding
- Solitary metastasis: colon, breast, renal, melanoma, osteosarcoma, testicular
Treatment
- Watchful waiting caveats
  - Every 3 months for 1st year and every 6 months for 2nd year
  - Tumors may not have constant growth
  - Small changes in growth in small nodules may be difficult to detect
- Benign nodules: None
- Needle biopsy
  - Useful for indeterminate nodules, need good cytopathologist
  - Pneumothorax rate 30%
- Malignancy
  - Resection: 5 yr survival up to 70% Stage I lung cancer

Selected References
1. Erasmus JJ et al: Solitary pulmonary nodules: Part I. Morphologic evaluation for differentiation of benign and malignant lesions. Radiographics 20:43-58, 2000
2. Erasmus JJ et al: Solitary pulmonary nodules: Part II. Evaluation of the indeterminate nodule. Radiographics 20:59-66, 2000
3. Swensen SJ et al: An integrated approach to evaluation of the solitary pulmonary nodule. Mayo Clin Proc 65:173-86, 1990

Metastases

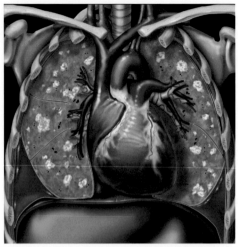

Diffuse bilateral varying sized nodules usually represent metastases. The differential diagnosis includes Wegeners, rheumatoid nodules, fungal pneumonia.

Key Facts
- Lung most common site of metastases: 50% at autopsy
- Thoracic sites for metastatic disease: Lung, pleura, bronchi
- Routes for spread: Hematogenous, endobronchial, lymphangitic, bronchogenic
- Variable-sized, sharply-defined, multiple pulmonary nodules
- CT sensitive but not specific for metastatic disease

Imaging Findings
General Features
- Best imaging clue: Variable sized sharply defined multiple pulmonary nodules

Chest Radiograph
- Hematogeneous patterns
  - Sharply-defined, variable-sized pulmonary nodules
  - Ill-defined margins seen in hemorrhagic metastases from choriocarcinoma
  - Preferentially distributed to lower lobes due to blood flow (gravity)
  - Cavitation with squamous or sarcoma cell type
  - Miliary pattern seen with medullary carcinoma thyroid, melanoma, renal cell, and ovarian carcinoma
  - Bone-forming tumors may calcify (osteogenic sarcoma, chondrosarcoma, thyroid) and may be ignored as granulomas
  - Occasionally complicated by pneumothorax especially from sarcomas
  - Solitary met: Renal cell, colon, breast, sarcomas, melanoma
- Lymphangitic pattern
  - Asymmetric nodular interstitial thickening
- Pleural pattern
  - Pleural effusion, may be massive, free or loculated
  - Discrete masses in pleura uncommon
- Endobronchial pattern

Metastases

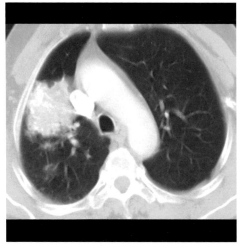

Chondrosarcoma metastases. Typical metastases has variable-sized, sharply defined pulmonary nodules. This metastases is atypical: Irregular margins and the mass contains foci of cartilagenous calcification. Bone or cartilage forming tumors may calcify.

- o Atelectasis, lobe or lung
- o Post-obstructive pneumonia
- Consolidative pattern
  - o Mimic pneumonia, peripheral consolidation with air-bronchograms
  - o Lipidic growth similar to bronchioloalveolar cell carcinoma
- Pulmonary embolus pattern
  - o Beaded enlarged vessels
  - o Pulmonary infarcts
- Bronchogenic spread
  - o Atelectasis
  - o Multifocal or diffuse consolidation
- Mediastinal spread: Mediastinal or hilar mass

CT Findings
- Hematogeneous nodules often have feeding artery ("cherry stem" appearance)
- Lymphangitic metastases characterized by peribronchial thickening or beaded septa
- Halo sign for hemorrhagic metastases
- Beaded enlarged vessels for intravascular growth, intravascular growth rare cause of tree-in-bud pattern
- Most metastases develop within outer 1/3 of the lung

Imaging Recommendations
- CT most sensitive examination and better characterizes pattern and extent of disease

Differential Diagnosis
AVMs
- Feeding arteries and draining veins

Metastases

Granulomas
- Calcified

Amyloid
- Calcified

Idiopathic Interstitial Pneumonia
- Septa not beaded, honeycombing

Pathology

General
- Pathology reflects metastatic route
- Epidemiology
  o Hematogeneous pattern typical tumors carcinomas (lung, breast, GI) and sarcomas
  o Lymphangitic pattern typically adenocarcinomas
  o Pleural pattern typically adenocarcinomas especially lung and breast
  o Consolidative pattern typical tumor adenocarcinoma GI tract, lymphoma
  o Pulmonary embolus pattern typical tumors hepatoma, breast, renal cell carcinoma, choriocarcinoma, angiosarcoma
  o Bronchogenic pattern typical tumors bronchioloalveolar cell carcinoma (consolidation), laryngotracheal papillomatosis (multiple cavitary nodules), basal cell carcinoma head and neck (endobronchial)
  o Mediastinal spread typical tumors nasopharyngeal, genitourinary (renal, prostate, testicular), breast
- Etiology-pathogenesis
  o Metastatic models
    ▪ Mechanical anatomic model: Metastases are filtered out in the first draining organ, commonly the lung
    ▪ Environmental model: Metastases preferentially find target sites due to favorable molecular or cellular environments, known as the "seed and soil" hypothesis

Gross Pathologic-Surgical Features
- Lipid growth, characteristic of BAC, uses the lung as scaffolding to grow
- Hilic growth, characteristic of hematogeneous mets, expand displace lung

Clinical Issues

Presentation
- Variable, depends on pattern of spread, may be asymptomatic

Natural History
- Germ cell metastases may evolve into benign teratomas which may then grow

Treatment
- Lung only site, consider resection, especially if interval from primary resection to metastases > 1 month

Prognosis
- Depends on histology of primary tumors, generally palliative radiation or chemotherapy

Selected References
1. Seo JB et al: Atypical pulmonary metastases: Spectrum of radiologic findings. Radiographics 21:403-17, 2001
2. Davis SD: CT evaluation for pulmonary metastases in patients with extrathoracic malignancy. Radiology 180:1-12, 1991

Septic, Venous Air Embolism

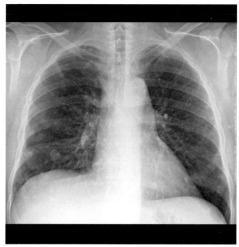

Multiple peripheral nodules appeared in a septic patient with Crohn's disease following pelvic abscess drainage.

Key Facts
- Septic emboli
  - Source: Tricuspid endocarditis, indwelling catheters
  - Peripheral wedge-shaped opacities from infarcts
  - Rapidly evolve and cavitate
- Venous air embolism
  - Source: Iatrogenic catheterization
  - Bell-shaped air in main pulmonary artery
  - Treatment: Left-lateral decubitus position

Imaging Findings
General Features
- Best imaging clue: Multiple patchy areas of consolidation rapidly evolving into cavitary nodules
Chest Radiograph
- Septic emboli
  - 1-3 cm peripheral nodular or wedge shaped opacities
  - Usually basilar (due to gravity and blood flow)
  - Evolve rapidly, cavitation common (50%)
    - Cavity wall usually thin
    - Lack air-fluid level
  - Often complicated by empyema
- Venous air embolism
  - Bell-shaped air collection main pulmonary artery
  - Edema
CT Findings
- Septic emboli
  - More sensitive than chest radiographs
  - Air bronchograms (25%)
  - Feeding vessel sign (66%)

Septic, Venous Air Embolism

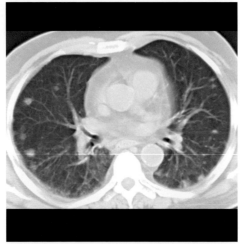

Multiple peripheral subpleural nodules several of which are fed by a pulmonary artery (cherry stem). None are cavitated. Diagnosis: Septic emboli. Blood cultures grew candida. Candida septic emboli rarely show cavitation.

- No intravascular clots
- Venous air embolism
  - More sensitive than chest radiography
  - Air in brachiocephalic veins in 25% after IV contrast administration

<u>Imaging Recommendations</u>
- Chest radiographs usually sufficient for diagnosis, CT may be useful in septic emboli

Differential Diagnosis
<u>Thromboemboli</u>
- Rare for venous emboli to cavitate

<u>Metastases</u>
- Metastases do not evolve rapidly

Pathology
<u>General</u>
- Septic emboli from infected embolic material
- Venous air emboli usually innocuous, if massive may give rise to Acute Respiratory Distress Syndrome (ARDS)
- Etiology pathogenesis
  - Venous air embolism
    - Foam formed from blood pulsating though air initiates coagulation

<u>Gross Pathologic-Surgical Features</u>
- Septic emboli: Necrotic infected lung
- Venous air emboli: Multiple fibrin clots in pulmonary arteries

<u>Microscopic Features</u>
- No specific features

Septic, Venous Air Embolism

Clinical Issues

Presentation

- Septic emboli
  - Source septic emboli
    - Indwelling venous catheters
    - Tricuspid endocarditis in IV drug abusers
    - Rarely pacemaker wires
  - Lemierre syndrome
    - Upper respiratory infection, immunocompetent host
    - Anaerobic infection
    - Septic phlebitis jugular vein
    - Septic emboli
    - ARDS
  - Staphylococcus aureus most common organism
  - Fever, cough, hemoptysis
  - Radiographic abnormalities may precede positive blood cultures
  - Often rupture into pleural space and result in empyema
- Venous air embolism
  - Source
    - Iatrogenic venous catheterization or IV contrast administration
    - Neurosurgical (head up position) procedures
    - Thoracic trauma
    - Scuba diving
    - Needle biopsy of the lung
  - Lethal dose 100-300 ml injected 100ml/sec
  - Air hunger, feeling of impending doom
  - "Mill-wheel" murmur

Treatment

- Septic emboli
  - Therapy with broad spectrum antibiotics
- Venous air embolism
  - Treatment to physically displace air from main pulmonary artery
    - Place patient in head down left-lateral decubitus position
    - Supportive oxygen
    - Hyperbaric oxygenation for severe cases

Selected References
1. Rossi SE et al: Nonthrombotic pulmonary emboli. AJR 174:1499-508, 2000
2. Kizer KW et al: Radiographic manifestations of venous air embolism. Radiology 144:35-9, 1982

Wegener's Granulomatosis

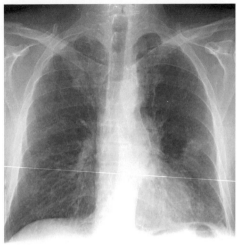

Wegener's granulomatosis. Ill-defined nodule left mid lung. Increased density left hilum. A characteristic feature not demonstrated in this case is subglottic stenosis.

Key Facts
- Vasculitis triad: Sinus, lung, renal disease
- Patterns: Cavitary nodules, focal consolidation, and diffuse edema
- Upper airway involvement may give rise to subglottic stenosis, recognizable but often overlooked on chest radiographs
- Therapy with corticosteroids and cyclophosphamide
- May relapse with same pattern or new pattern typically airway stenosis or consolidation

Imaging Findings
<u>General Features</u>
- Best imaging clue: Multiple cavitary nodules and subglottic stenosis
<u>Chest Radiograph</u>
- Single or multiple nodules
  - Sharp or ill-defined (depends on surrounding hemorrhage)
  - Frequently thick-walled cavitation (50%)
  - Rapid expansion suggests superinfection or hemorrhage
  - Variable size, may coalesce into large masses
  - Preferentially lower lobes
  - May be unilateral (15%)
  - When multiple usually < 10
  - May spontaneously regress
- Focal or multifocal consolidation, also may cavitate
- Diffuse consolidation due to hemorrhage (25%)
- Interstitial pattern rare, usually a sequel of hemorrhage or edema in patients with cardiac or renal involvement but can also be due to granulomas
- Pleural effusions (20%)
- Hilar or mediastinal adenopathy rare
- Subglottic stenosis (more common in women) later in course of disease

Wegener's Granulomatosis

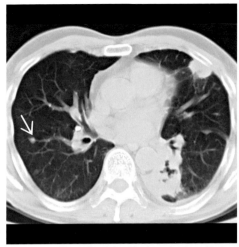

Wegener's. Multiple variable sized nodules. The irregular shaped lesion in the medial left base is partially cavitated. Note the vascular connection to the nodule in the right mid-lung (arrow).

- More peripheral airway stenosis may result in atelectasis (lobar or segmental)
- Post-therapy
  - Parenchymal findings should start to clear within 1 week
    - If no improvement, suspect superinfection
  - Complete normalization averages 1 month (2-6 weeks)
- Relapse
  - 50% have same pattern and location
  - Otherwise relapse typically airway stenosis or consolidative pattern

CT Findings
- Nodules preferentially subpleural peripheral location
- Like metastases, nodules may have feeding vessel
- Peripheral wedge-shaped consolidation probably due to infarcts
- Nodules may demonstrate halo sign due to surrounding hemorrhage
- Bronchi concentrically thickened, either focal or long segments

Imaging Recommendations
- CT more sensitive, chest radiographs usually sufficient for diagnosis and therapy

Differential Diagnosis

Metastases
- History of squamous cell or sarcoma malignancy

Infections, Fungal and Tuberculosis
- Identical radiographic findings, culture required to exclude

Septic Emboli
- Nodules rapidly evolve

Lymphomatoid Granulomatosis (Non-Hodgkin's Lymphoma)
- CNS or skin disease, otherwise multiple cavitary nodules identical

Rheumatoid Necrobiotic Nodules
- History of joint disease

Wegener's Granulomatosis

Pulmonary-Renal Syndromes
- Goodpastures
- Hemosiderosis
- Periarteritis nodosa
- Churg-Strauss syndrome
- Lymphomatoid granulomatosis
- Systemic lupus erythematosus

Pathology
General
- Pulmonary vasculitis: Inflammation and necrosis of blood vessels
  o Lung commonly involved in systemic vasculitis due to large vascular bed and exposure to airway antigens
- Etiology-pathogenesis: Unknown, suspect inhaled antigen
- Epidemiology
  o Prevalence 3:100,000, slightly more frequent in men, 40-50 years of age
Microscopic Features
- Vasculitis small and medium-sized vessels, necrosis, hemorrhage common
- Non-necrotizing granulomas (must exclude infection)

Clinical Issues
Presentation
- Usually related to upper respiratory tract: Sinusitis and rhinitis
- Pulmonary symptoms nonspecific
  o Cough, fever, dyspnea, hemoptysis, chest pain
  o Those with nodules less likely to have symptoms
- Frequency of systemic involvement
  o Lung (95%), upper airway (85%), renal (80%), skin (50%), joints (50%), cardiac (30%), CNS (20%), eye (20%)
- Limited: Lung only, usually evolves into systemic disease
- Serum c-ANCA (cytoplasmic antineutrophil cytoplasmic autoantibody)
  o Sensitivity 95% classic disease, 70% limited disease, specificity 99%
  o Important in diagnosis, levels correlate with disease activity
- Lung or renal biopsy for diagnosis
Natural History
- Delayed diagnosis, consolidation usually ascribed to infection, diffuse hemorrhage nonspecific, recognition dependent on systemic nature of disease
Treatment
- Steroids and immunosuppressive drugs (particularly cyclophosphamide)
- Cytotoxic therapy predisposes to superinfection
Prognosis
- Renal disease most common cause of death

Selected References
1. Frazier AA et al: Pulmonary angiitis and granulomatosis: Radiologic-pathologic correlation. Radiographics 18:687-710, 1998
2. Aberle DR et al: Thoracic manifestations of Wegener granulomatosis: Diagnosis and course. Radiology 174:703-9, 1990

Arteriovenous Malformations

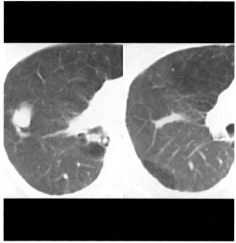

Arteriovenous malformation (AVM). Contiguous CT images through right upper lobe nodule. Lobulated nodule has large draining vein which can be traced back to the hilum.

Key Facts
- Majority associated with hereditary hemorrhagic telangiectasia (HHT)
- Single or multiple pulmonary nodules with feeding arteries and draining veins
- CT most sensitive study to screen for pulmonary arteriovenous malformations (AVM)
- Treatment recommended for AVMs with > 3 mm diameter feeding artery
- Treatment intravascular embolotherapy
- Persistent AVM 1 month after embolotherapy suggests failure

Imaging Findings
General Features
- Best imaging clue: Lobulated nodule with feeding artery and draining vein
Chest Radiograph
- Lobulated, sharply-defined solitary pulmonary nodule (SPN) connected to feeding vessel(s) and draining vein
- May be multiple
- May have rim calcification
- 70% located in lower lobes
- Increase in size with Valsalva maneuver
- Infarcts may develop after embolotherapy
  - More common with peripheral AVMs
  - Often heralded by pleurisy and pleural effusion
CT Findings
- Procedure of choice to screen for AVMs
- More sensitive than pulmonary angiography
- Useful to plan embolotherapy
- After embocotherapy < 1 month
  - 2/3 disappear or shrink
  - 1/3 same size

Arteriovenous Malformations

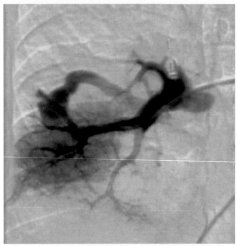

Digital subtraction angiogram. Simple AVM supplied by single artery and draining vein. Angiograms rarely done now for diagnosis but therapy with balloon occlusion.

- • Because either thrombosed or persistent perfusion
- Post embolotherapy after 1 month
  - o If same size suspect embolization failure due to persistent perfusion

<u>MRI Findings</u>
- MR angiography similar to CT for detection
- 99mTc-labelled macroaggregates may be used to estimate size of right to left shunt by measuring activity accumulation in kidney (normally macroaggregates will not pass through pulmonary capillary bed)

<u>Imaging Recommendations</u>
- CT most sensitive examination for detection, useful to plan therapy

Differential Diagnosis
<u>Carcinoid</u>
- May enhance at CT, no connecting artery or vein

<u>Metastases</u>
- May have feeding vessels at CT, these are not identified on chest radiographs and are much smaller than the feeding arteries of AVMs and metastases also do not have large draining veins

<u>SPN</u>
- In differential to SPN, only AVM has feeding artery and vein

Pathology
<u>General</u>
- Congenital communications between artery and vein
- Etiology and pathogenesis
  - o Right to left shunt
  - o Hypoxemia uncorrected with 100% O_2
- Epidemiology
  - o Multiple AVMs highly associated with HHT (90%)
  - o Conversely 10% of patients with HHT have AVMs

Arteriovenous Malformations

Gross Pathologic-Surgical Features
- Simple and complex
  - Simple: One feeding artery, one aneurysm, one draining vein
  - Complex more than one feeding artery

Clinical Issues
Presentation
- Usually become symptomatic 40-60 years of age
- Epistaxis presenting feature due to HHT associated nasal telangiectasia
- Asymptomatic to dyspnea, cyanosis and clubbing depending on size of shunt
- Neurologic events: TIAs and stroke in 20-40% due to loss of lung filter
- Hypoxemia exaggerated in upright position (orthodeoxia) due to increased shunting in lower lobe AVMs
- May lead to high output CHF
Treatment
- Intravascular coils or balloons
  - Treat all AVMs with feeding artery > 3 mm in diameter
- Complications
  - Paradoxical embolization of coils or balloons
    - More common with simple than complex AVM
  - Infarction
    - More common with distal than central occlusion
Prognosis
- Recurrence possible but rare, periodic screening CT (every 5 years)
- Family members should be screened for HHT

Selected References
1. Remy J et al: Pulmonary arteriovenous malformations: Evaluation with CT of the chest before and after treatment. Radiology 182:809-16, 1992
2. Remy-Jardin M et al: Transcatheter occlusion of pulmonary arterial circulation and collateral supply: Failures, incidents, and complications. Radiology 180: 699-705, 1991

PocketRadiologist™
Chest
Top 100 Diagnoses

PLEURA

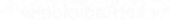

Pleural Effusions

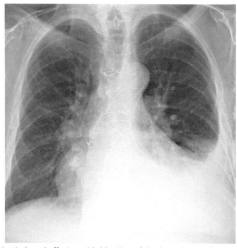

Moderate sized pleural effusion with blunting of the lateral costophrenic angle. Free fluid has smooth sharp meniscus.

Key Facts
- Pleural effusions common, fluid analysis essential for differentiation
- Normal pleural fluid quantity 5 ml, lateral decubitus will detect 10 ml
- Large effusions may invert hemidiaphragm and impair ventilation
- Radiographic methods poor to separate transudates from exudates

Imaging Findings
General Features
- Best imaging clue: Blunting costophrenic angles
Chest Radiograph
- Sequence of accumulation upright film: Subpulmonic > posterior angle > lateral angle
- Subpulmonic
  - Flattening and "elevation" of hemidiaphragm
  - Lateral shift of diaphragm apex
  - Separation of gastric bubble from diaphragm (normal < 1.5 cm)
  - On lateral: Diaphragm flat anteriorly then sharply descends at major fissure
- Posterior costophrenic sulcus (only lateral view)
  - Blunting posterior costophrenic sulcus
  - Average quantity needed to blunt: 50 ml
- Lateral costophrenic sulcus (only PA view)
  - Blunting lateral costophrenic sulcus
  - Average quantity needed to blunt: 200 ml
- Inversion hemidiaphragm
  - Medial displacement of gastric air bubble
  - Seen with large effusions greater than 2000 ml
  - Chest fluoroscopy to demonstrate paradoxical respiration (pendelluft)
    - Inspiration: Inverted diaphragm ascends
    - Expiration: Inverted diaphragm descends

Pleural Effusions

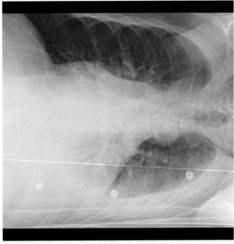

Lateral decubitus is the most sensitive radiographic exam to demonstrate pleural fluid. As little as 10 ml can be detected (normal is 5 ml). Generally safe to do blind percutaneous thoracentesis if layered fluid > 1 cm thick.

- Supine film poorest examination to detect fluid
  - Sensitivity 70%, up to 500 ml must accumulate for reliable detection
  - Generalized increase in density hemithorax, meniscus often absent
  - Apical cap (apex most dependent portion of supine hemithorax)
- Fissural accumulation helpful finding for the presence of small effusions
  - May preferentially accumulate air or fluid in COPD patients
  - Minor fissure pseudotumor may be mistaken for pulmonary mass
  - Fluid in incomplete major fissure pitfall for pneumothorax or pneumomediastinum
    - Fluid in fissure has curvilinear edge concave toward hilum
- Rapid accumulation suggests torn thoracic duct, perforated vein by central venous catheter, esophageal rupture, trauma, malignancy

CT Findings
- No reliable distinction between exudates and transudates
- Pleural effusion vs. ascites
  - Pleural fluid peripheral, ascites central
  - Pleural fluid displaces crus anteriorly
  - Pleural fluid posterior to bare area, spared with ascites
  - Pleural fluid interface with liver or spleen indistinct, sharp with ascites
  - Pitfall: Findings reversed for inverted diaphragm
    - Pleural fluid central, ascites peripheral
    - Pleural fluid will get progressively smaller with caudal progression

Ultrasound
- Echoic effusions usually associated with exudates
- Anechoic effusions may be either transudates or exudates (50%)

Imaging Recommendations
- Lateral decubitus examination will detect as little as 10 ml of fluid
- US useful for thoracentesis guidance
- CT for complex disease

Pleural Effusions

Differential Diagnosis
Elevated Diaphragm
- Costophrenic angles sharp, apex not shifted laterally

Pathology
General
- Pleural effusion, common sign from cardiopulmonary disease or reaction to diseases located adjacent to the hemidiaphragm (pancreas, liver, etc.)
- Etiology-pathogenesis
  - Starling forces (transudates) or inflammation (exudates)
  - Exudate, simple
    - Pleural fluid: Serum protein ratio > 0.5 or LDH ratio > 0.6
    - Pleural fluid LDH > 200 IU or protein > 3 gm/dl
  - Exudate, complicated
    - PH < 7.2, LDH > 1000, Glucose < 60 mg/dl
    - Positive Gram stain
  - Transudates commonly due to CHF, uremia, hypoalbuminemia (< 1.5 gm/dl) or myxedema
  - Exudates commonly due to infection, infarction, malignancy
  - Chylothorax, milky appearance (50%) may be bloody
    - 2000 ml cloudy, odorless and sterile
    - Triglycerides > 100 mg/dl, chylomicrons present
    - Causes: Trauma or surgery, lymphoma, LAM, congenital, idiopathic
Gross Pathologic-Surgical Features
- Normal pleural fluid volume approximately 5 ml total (2.5 / hemithorax)
- Normal pleura surface area 2000 cm^2
- Normally no communication between pleural spaces

Clinical Issues
Presentation
- Nonspecific symptoms if present: Cough, chest pain, dyspnea
- D'Amato sign
  - Displacement in dullness from vertebral area to cardiac region when patient moves from sitting to lateral decubitus position (due to free pleural effusion)
- Asymptomatic effusions common due to CHF, postop, malignancy, post-partum, benign asbestos effusion, uremia, tuberculosis
Treatment
- Thoracentesis
  - Blind tap safe for fluid > 1 cm thickness lateral decubitus examination
- Chest tube drainage for complicated exudates or symptomatic effusions
- Thoracic duct tear
  - Diet medium-chain triglycerides (absorbed into portal system)
  - Surgical ligation of thoracic duct for persistent drainage (> 2 weeks)

Selected References
1. Müller NL: Imaging of the pleura. Radiology 186:297-309, 1993
2. Raasch BN et al: Pleural effusion: Explanation of some typical appearances. AJR 139:899-904, 1982

Pleural Thickening

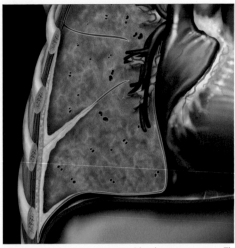

Diffuse smooth pleural thickening may occur with asbestos exposure. The differential diagnosis includes mesothelioma, metastatic pleural disease, and fibrothorax following remote infection or hemothorax.

Key Facts
- Fibrothorax may follow trauma, empyema, or asbestos exposure
- Fibrothorax may give rise to rounded atelectasis or trapped lung
- Split calcified pleura may represent dormant empyema
- New pleural thickening over pre-existing cavities suggests aspergilloma
- Aggressive fibromatosis produces locally invasive large chest wall mass
- Apical caps, normal process of aging

Imaging Findings
Chest Radiograph
- Diffuse pleural thickening
  - Extent > 1/4 of chest wall
  - Margins sharp in profile, indistinct en face
  - May be seen in only 1 view (frontal or lateral)
- Fibrothorax
  - Diffuse or focal pleural thickening
  - Associated upper lobe lung abnormalities suggest tuberculous empyema
  - Associated bilateral pleural abnormalities suggest asbestos-related disease
  - Associated with multiple rib fractures suggest traumatic hemothorax
  - Complications
    - Round atelectasis: Peripheral mass adjacent to pleural thickening
    - Pleural peel traps lung and prevents its expansion
- Dormant tuberculous empyema
  - Lenticular shape
  - Calcification both parietal and visceral pleura
  - > 2 cm separation between calcified layers
  - Adjacent ribs often enlarged due to chronic periostitis

Pleural Thickening

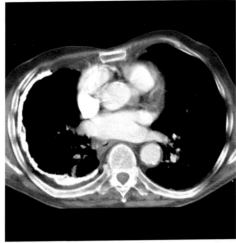

Calcific fibrothorax may be due to old empyema, hemorrhage, or infection (especially tuberculosis). Pleural process is restrictive decreasing volume in the affected hemithorax. Note the proliferation of extrapleural fat adjacent to the calcification. This finding signifies both chronicity and a benign process.

- o May evolve into empyema necessitatis or bronchopleural fistula
- Aspergillus superinfection
  - o New pleural thickening adjacent to pre-existing cavitary disease
  - o Aspergilloma may not be radiographically evident
  - o Aspergilloma usually can be identified at CT
- Asbestos diffuse pleural thickening
  - o Blunts costophrenic angle
    - ▪ Pleural plaques unusual in this location
  - o Secondary to benign asbestos effusion
- Apical cap
  - o Sharp, smooth or undulating margin
  - o Usually < 5 mm thick
  - o Unilateral or bilateral
    - ▪ Right > left
  - o Incidence increases with age
- Aggressive fibromatosis (desmoid)
  - o Large chest wall mass
  - o May destroy ribs

CT Findings
- More sensitive than chest radiography to identify pleural thickening and pleural calcification
- Examination of choice to evaluate complex pleural disease
- Extrapleural fat often hypertrophied from chronic pleural disease
- Lack of superimposition ideal to identify associated parenchymal changes
- Aggressive fibromatosis may enhance with intravenous contrast
- Curvilinear course of blood vessels into round atelectasis (comet tail sign) better demonstrated at CT

Pleural Thickening

Differential Diagnosis

Metastases or Mesothelioma
- Circumferential thickening
- Nodular pleural thickening
- Parietal pleural thickening > 1 cm thickness
- Mediastinal pleural involvement

Fibrous Tumor of Pleura
- May change location with position

Askin Tumor
- Young adults, often extends into rib or chest-wall

Lipoma or Extrapleural Fat
- Fat density at CT

Pathology

General
- Fibrothorax nonspecific healed response to infection or inflammation
- Etiology-pathogenesis
  o Aggressive fibromatosis
    ▪ Site related to previous trauma or surgery
    ▪ Associated conditions: Gardner's syndrome, pregnancy, estrogen medications
  o Apical cap
    ▪ Normal process of aging
    ▪ May be related to ischemia
    ▪ Normally PA pressure just sufficient to get blood to lung apex
    ▪ Age 40: 5%
    ▪ Age 70: 50%

Gross Pathologic-Surgical Features
- Lung apex normally covered by thicker fascia (Sibson's fascia)

Microscopic Features
- Fibrothorax: Nonspecific collagen and fibrosis
- Asbestos fibers in asbestos related disease
- Aggressive fibromatosis
  o Well-differentiated fibroblasts in collagen matrix
  o No malignant features

Clinical Issues

Presentation
- Dormant empyema, usually asymptomatic finding discovered incidentally on chest radiographs

Treatment & Prognosis
- Dormant empyema
  o Antituberculous drugs, consider surgical resection
- Aggressive fibromatosis wide resections, local recurrence frequent (50%)
- Trapped lung
  o Long term drainage of empyema
  o Surgical decortication

Selected References
1. Müller NL: Imaging of the pleura. Radiology 186:297-309, 1993
2. Leung AN et al: CT in differential diagnosis of diffuse pleural disease. AJR 154:487-92, 1990

Asbestos Related Pleural Disease

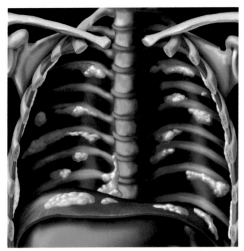

Asbestos related pleural plaques occur primarily on the parietal pleura and diaphragms, sparing the costophrenic angles and mediastinal pleura. They are < 10 mm in thickness, often calcify and do not cause restrictive lung disease.

Key Facts
- Pleural effusion earliest manifestation of asbestos exposure
- Pleural plaque marker for previous asbestos exposure
- Short asbestos fibers migrate from lung into pleura, entrapped along parietal stomas
- Pleural plaque latency 20-30 years
- Diffuse pleural thickening may be due to previous asbestos effusion

Imaging Findings
<u>General Features</u>
- Best imaging clue: Multiple calcified diaphragmatic pleural plaques
<u>Chest Radiograph</u>
- Benign pleural effusion
  - Small to moderate, unilateral or bilateral
  - Often recurs, eventually spontaneously resolve over 6-month period
- Pleural plaque
  - Location
    - Posterolateral and anterolateral chest wall (oblique films more likely bring them into profile)
    - Central tendon diaphragm
  - Relative symmetrical involvement
    - Left hemithorax more involved than right
  - 2–15 mm thick
  - Sharp borders in profile, shaped like a butte
  - Rarely extend more than 4 rib interspaces
  - Spares apices and costophrenic angle
  - Linear calcification in profile, holly leaf calcification en face
  - Sensitivity of radiographs for plaques: 30%, false positives 40%

Asbestos Related Pleural Disease

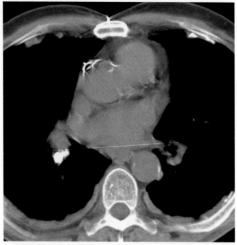

Asbestos pleural plaques. Multiple pleural plaques. Individual plaques are butte shaped. Calcification may be diffuse, linear or punctate. Typically more plaques found in the dorsal aspect of the hemithorax and central tendon.

- Diffuse pleural thickening
  - Previous benign asbestos effusion (50%)
  - Covers more than 1/4 of chest wall
  - May also represent numerous confluent individual plaques
  - Usually involves the costophrenic angle
  - Unilateral or bilateral
  - May progressively worsen

CT Findings
- More sensitive for pleural plaques, differentiates plaque from fat, muscle or other mimics

Imaging Recommendations
- CT useful to investigate focal pleural abnormalities

Differential Diagnosis

Subpleural Fat
- Symmetric, mid-lateral chest wall 4th to 8th ribs
- May extend into fissure
- Associated with other fat deposition: Pericardial fat pads, widened mediastinum, thickened chest wall
- No calcification

Serratus Anterior Muscle
- Symmetric mid chest wall
- Between intercostal spaces
- Triangular in shape
- Edge fades inferiorly
- No calcification

Rib Fractures
- Abnormal rib contour, posterolateral location

Mesothelioma
- Associated with pleural plaques

Asbestos Related Pleural Disease

- Unilateral rind pleural thickening shrinks ipsilateral hemithorax

Metastatic Adenocarcinoma
- Lobulated unilateral pleural thickening in patient with known malignancy

Previous Hemothorax
- Unilateral, multiple healed rib fractures

Previous Empyema
- Adjacent lung abnormal, scarring from previous pneumonia

Pathology
General
- Pleural plaques have no propensity to degenerate into malignancy
- Etiology-pathogenesis
  - Short fibers transported from lung into pleura
  - Migrate to parietal pleural stoma
  - Trapped in stoma, long-term low-grade inflammation

Gross Pathologic-Surgical Features
- Acellular, white, smooth, subpleural collections of collagen
- Geographic shape
- Adhesion between visceral and parietal pleural absent

Microscopic Features
- Collagen in basket weave pattern
- Calcification in 85%
- Extent and thickness correlate with asbestos bodies

Clinical Issues
Presentation
- Benign pleural effusion
  - 2/3 asymptomatic, 1/3 fever, pleuritic chest pain, dyspnea
- Pleural plaque
  - Asymptomatic, no impairment of pulmonary function
  - Also associated with cigarette smoking
  - Associated with chrysotile asbestos
  - 25% with asbestosis have no plaques
  - 90% with mesothelioma have no plaques
  - Slight increased risk of lung cancer in smokers
- Diffuse pleural thickening impairs ventilation
  - SOB, dyspnea on exertion
  - Restrictive pulmonary function tests

Natural History
- Benign pleural effusion earliest asbestos manifestation: 10 years after exposure, latent period may be decades, typically last 6 months but maybe as long as a decade
- Pleural plaque 20-30 year latent period

Treatment & Prognosis
- Smoking cessation
- Lung cancer screening should be considered

Selected References
1. Lynch DA et al: Conventional and high resolution computed tomography in the diagnosis of asbestos-related diseases. Radiographics 9:523-51, 1989
2. Herbert A: Pathogenesis of pleurisy, pleural fibrosis, and mesothelial proliferation. Thorax 41:176-89, 1986

Pneumothorax

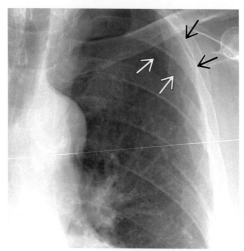

Moderate sized pneumothorax. Fracture left 5th rib. The visceral pleura (white arrows) is paper thin. Note: The difference between the visceral pleura line (white arrows) and the normal extrapleural line (black arrows).

Key Facts
- Height main risk factor for primary (spontaneous) pneumothorax
- Secondary associated with trauma and diffuse lung disease
- Air reabsorbed from pleural space at rate of 1.5% day
- Supine film less sensitive than upright film for pneumothorax
- Common pleural space (buffalo chest) uncommon
- Common clinical rule: Pneumothorax larger than 25% requires chest tube drainage

Imaging Findings
Chest Radiograph
- High sensitivity, expiratory film rarely needed
- Visceral pleural line usually parallels chest wall
- Supine, less sensitive (70%)
  - Deep sulcus (anterolateral hemithorax most nondependent in supine position)
  - Relative transradiancy hemithorax
  - Mediastinal contours or heart border sharper than uninvolved side
  - Visualization pericardial tags or fat pads which become "mass like"
  - Air in minor fissure
- Tension
  - Contralateral mediastinal shift
  - Ipsilateral depression diaphragm
  - Collapsed lung
  - Expansion rib cage
  - Pneumothorax usually large
    - If lungs stiff from ARDS, small pneumothorax may produce tension
- Subpulmonic pneumothorax
  - Unusual location, may be seen in COPD

Pneumothorax

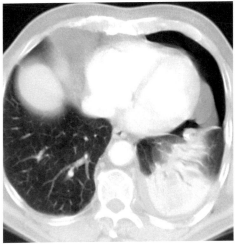

Large pneumothorax. Lower lobe contusion. In this example there would be no visceral pleural line on the chest radiography as the lung extends to the chest wall in the supine position.

- Pneumothorax ex vacuo
  - Collection of air in pleural space adjacent to collapsed lobe
  - May resolve with reexpansion of lobe
  - Considered a vacuum joint phenomenon
  - Conversely a large pneumothorax may collapse an upper lobe due to bronchial kinking from weight of the lung, lobe will reexpand with chest tube drainage

CT Findings
- More sensitive than chest radiography for free air
- More sensitive than chest radiography for apical blebs (85%)

Differential Diagnosis

Skin Edge, Scapula, Hair, Extraneous Monitoring or Support Lines
- An edge rather than a line, often extends outside chest wall
  - Edge thicker and fades off medially compared to visceral line

Bullae
- Air will not change location with position
- No visceral pleural line

Pathology

General
- Congenital
  - Pneumothorax associated with connective tissue disorders: Marfan's; Ehlers-Danlos, cutis laxa, pseudoxanthoma elasticum
- Etiology-pathogenesis
  - Patients height risk factor for spontaneous pneumothorax, tall lung may be subject to more gravitational stress
  - Secondary to underlying condition
    - COPD

Pneumothorax

- Interstitial lung disease, especially alveolar sarcoid, LAM and Langerhans cell histiocytosis
- Catamenial
- Traumatic
- Neoplastic, especially sarcoma metastases
- Post-infectious pneumatoceles (PCP or Staph aureus)

Gross Pathologic-Surgical Features
- Subpleural apical blebs or paraseptal emphysema commonly identified at CT in patients with spontaneous pneumothorax
- Humans have separate pleural space for each lung
  - Transient communication immediately after median sternotomy
  - Long term communication in heart-lung transplants
  - Unilateral insult will result in bilateral pneumothorax, known as buffalo chest (buffalo normally have common pleural space about both lungs)
  - Single chest tube will drain both pleural spaces

Microscopic Features
- Free air may induce eosinophils within pleural fluid

Clinical Issues
Presentation
- Chest pain, dyspnea, may be asymptomatic

Treatment
- Chest tube drainage common for pneumothorax > 25%
  - Size less important than patient's physiologic status
  - Small pneumothorax significant in patients with little reserve (COPD)
  - Large pneumothorax may not be significant in young patient with large respiratory reserve
  - Absorption of air in pleural space: 1.5% per day
    - Increased with use of supplemental oxygen
  - Re-expansion pulmonary edema (< 1%)
    - Develops within hours of drainage
    - Transient, resolves over several days
    - More likely with large chronic pleural space collections
  - Failure to expand lung may be due to chest tube malposition, underlying tracheal, bronchial, or esophageal tear, or due to trapped lung with pleural metastases
- Pleurodesis, chemical for recurrent spontaneous pneumothorax
- Surgical pleurodesis and bullectomy for refractory or recurrent pneumothorax

Selected References
1. Collins CD et al: Quantification of pneumothorax size on chest radiographs using interpleural distances: Regression analysis based on volume measurements from helical CT. AJR 165:1127-30, 1995
2. Greene R et al: Pneumothorax. Semin Roentgenol 12:313-25, 1977

Malignant Mesothelioma

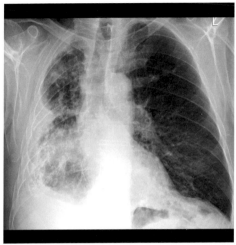

Malignant mesothelioma. Diffuse lobulated pleural thickening right hemithorax. Thickening extends into the fissure. Entire right hemithorax is small, a characteristic feature of malignant mesothelioma.

Key Facts
- Rare pleural tumor associated with asbestos exposure
- Long, thin asbestos fibers more likely to induce mesothelioma
- Pleural effusion near universal, may be only manifestation
- Diffuse nodular pleural thickening, small hemithorax
- Poor prognosis: 12 month median survival

Imaging Findings
Chest Radiograph
- Pleural effusion (95%), may be only finding
- Lobulated pleural thickening
- Hemithorax usually small
  - Sometimes expanded due to massive pleural effusion
- Pleural plaques in uninvolved hemithorax (5%)

CT Findings
- Surgical decisions depend on chest wall, diaphragmatic, and mediastinal involvement
  - CT sensitive but not specific for invasion, surgery necessary unless gross involvement detected
- Gravitational distribution
  - Tumor thicker at base
- Contralateral pleural plaques 10%
- Nodal disease difficult to evaluate
- Tendency to extend along needle or chest tube drainage tract (20%)
- Diffuse hepatic calcification may be seen with liver metastases

MR Findings
- Coronal imaging useful to evaluate transdiaphragmatic extent

Imaging Recommendations
- CT to evaluate nature and extent of pleural disease

Malignant Mesothelioma

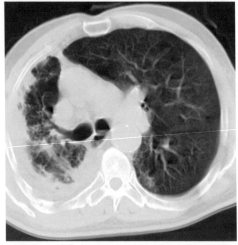

Malignant mesothelioma. Lobulated pleural thickening completely encases the right lung. Linear atelectasis in the right mid and lower lung.

Differential Diagnosis
General Separation Benign vs. Malignant Pleural Disease
- Favors malignancy: Circumferential involvement, nodular pleural thickening, parietal pleura > 1 cm thick, mediastinal involvement

Metastatic Adenocarcinoma
- May not have pleural effusion (50%)
- Shrinkage of hemithorax less common with metastatic adenocarcinoma
- Visceral pleura rather than parietal pleura

Empyema
- Rarely involves the entire pleural space

Thymoma
- Anterior mediastinal mass, discreet pleural masses

Lymphoma
- Other nodal disease, usually secondary to known disease

Asbestos Pleural Disease
- Benign effusions diagnosis of exclusion

Tuberculosis
- Parenchymal changes in upper lobes

Hemangioendothelioma
- Rare, older men
- Pleural thickening not as extensive

Pathology
General
- Etiology-Pathogenesis
  - Asbestos fiber induction depends on fiber aspect ratio (length:width)
    - Higher aspect ratio the higher the prevalence of mesothelioma
    - Crocidolite > amosite > chrysotile (rarely causes mesothelioma)
  - Dose response relationship, latent period from exposure 30–45 yrs
    - Exposure may be incidental
- Epidemiology

Malignant Mesothelioma

- o Rare tumor, 10/1,000,000 men, typically 50-70 years of age
- o Prevalence depends on exposed population
  - ▪ 5% insulation workers die of mesothelioma

Gross Pathologic-Surgical Features
- Primarily involves parietal pleura, rapidly involves the entire ipsilateral pleura

Microscopic Features
- Three histologic types
  - o Epithelial (50%); best prognosis
  - o Sarcomatous (20%)
  - o Biphasic (both cell types) (30%)

Staging
- Stages I – IV
  - o I: (20%)
    - ▪ Ia: Ipsilateral parietal pleural, no involvement visceral pleura
    - ▪ Ib: Ipsilateral parietal and visceral pleura
  - o II: (50%)
    - ▪ Involvement of diaphragm muscle or extension into lung
  - o III: (25%)
    - ▪ Any nodal involvement or primary tumor with limited extension into chest wall, mediastinal fat, pericardium
  - o IV: (< 5%)
    - ▪ Contralateral mediastinal nodes, primary tumor into vital mediastinal structure, through diaphragm or pericardium or extensive (unresectable chest wall involvement) or distant metastases
- Potentially resectable: Stage I-III

Clinical Issues
Presentation
- Chest pain, dyspnea, fever, and weight loss
- Pleural fluid
  - o Bloody (30%)
  - o Glucose decreased
  - o Hyaluronic acid increased
- Course often complicated by thrombophlebitis

Treatment
- Extrapleural pneumonectomy
- Palliative radiation therapy or chemotherapy
- Local radiation prophylactic to chest wall needle tracts

Prognosis
- Dismal, median survival 12 months

Selected References
1. Patz EF Jr. et al: The proposed new international TNM staging system for malignant pleural mesothelioma: Application to imaging. AJR 166:323-7, 1996
2. Miller BH et al: From the archives of the AFIP. Malignant pleural mesothelioma: Radiologic-pathologic correlation. Radiographics 16:613-44, 1996

Fibrous Tumor Of The Pleura

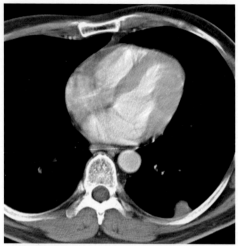

Localized fibrous tumor of the pleura. Small broad-based pleural or lung mass in the posterior left hemithorax. Although fibrous tumors may be mobile, most are sessile.

Key Facts
- Synonyms: Benign mesothelioma
- Not related to asbestos exposure
- Large, pedunculated, peripheral tumor
- Classic but rare symptoms hypoglycemia and hypertrophic osteoarthropathy
- Malignant lesions (20%) associated with calcification or pleural effusion
- Tend to recur locally, require long-term surveillance

Imaging Findings
General Features
- Best imaging clue: Peripheral mass changes location with position
Chest Radiograph
- Peripheral, lobulated, sharply-marginated mass
- Lenticular shape, longitudinal axis parallels chest wall
- Variable sized usually > 7 cm
- Pedunculated lesions change location with position
- Pleural effusions 20% (more common with malignant lesions)
CT Findings
- Characteristic obtuse angle of pleural lesions absent
- Calcification 5% (more common with malignant lesions)
- No chest wall involvement
- Enhance with contrast
- Large tumors inhomogeneous due to collagen and cystic degeneration
MRI Findings
- Low T_1 and Low T_2 due to fibrous content
Imaging Recommendations
- CT useful to characterize pleural abnormalities

Fibrous Tumor Of The Pleura

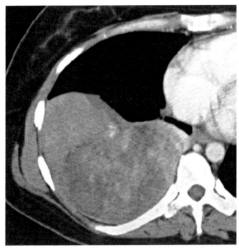

Large heterogenous mass filling nearly 50% of the right hemithorax. Large lesions are more apt to be mobile or associated with hypoglycemia and hypertrophic osteoarthropathy.

Differential Diagnosis
<u>Pleural Lipomas</u>
- Fat density, may be pedunculated and change position

<u>Diaphragmatic Hernias</u>
- Bowel contents or mesenteric fat, may change position

<u>Fibrin Ball</u>
- Smaller "pea sized", free in pleural space and may change position

Pathology
<u>General</u>
- 2/3 visceral pleura, 1/3 parietal
- Parietal origin more likely malignant
- Etiology-pathogenesis
  - No asbestos association
- Epidemiology
  - No gender preference
  - Age 45-60

<u>Gross Surgical-Pathologic Features</u>
- Pleural heterogeneous soft-tissue mass
- Pedicle 50%, signifies benignity
- 20% malignant
  - May have calcification

<u>Microscopic Features</u>
- Patternless
  - Fibroblasts and connective tissue in random pattern
- Hemangiopericytoma
  - Irregular branching capillaries and vessels

Fibrous Tumor Of The Pleura

Clinical Issues

<u>Presentation</u>
- Asymptomatic 25%
- Cough, chest pain, dyspnea
- Large tumors > 10 cm associated with
  - Hypertrophic osteoarthropathy or
  - Hypoglycemia (5%)

<u>Treatment & Prognosis</u>
- Surgical excision
- Benign tumors tend to recur years later (15%)
  - Require long-term surveillance

Selected References
1. Lee KS et al: CT findings in benign fibrous mesothelioma of the pleura: Pathologic correlation in nine patients. AJR 158: 983-6, 1992
2. England DM et al: Localized benign and malignant fibrous tumors of the pleura. A clinicopathologic review of 223 cases. Am J Surg Pathol 13:640-58, 1989

Benign Pleural Mass

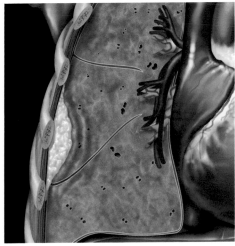

Pleural or extrapleural fat can change shape with respiration or position. Fatty attenuation (-30 to -100 HU) with CT is diagnostic.

Key Facts
- Pleural lesions: Radiographic characteristics change on orthogonal views
- Lipoma most common benign tumor of the pleura
  - Any soft tissue (other than linear strands) should suggest liposarcoma
- Fibrin balls loose within pleural space, follow exudative effusions
- Splenosis follows trauma to spleen and diaphragm multiple left-sided pleural masses

Imaging Findings
Chest Radiograph
- Pleural mass
  - Sharp margin in profile
  - Indistinct margin en face
  - Different radiographic characteristics in orthogonal views
  - Homogeneous
  - Convex to lung
  - Obtuse angle to chest wall
  - Consecutive examinations may have different radiographic characteristics due to slight changes in obliquity (changing tangential margins)
- Lipoma
  - Oval or lenticular shaped
  - May grow slowly
  - Large lesions may be pedunculated and change location with positional maneuvers
  - Smaller lesions may change shape with respiration (lipomas are soft)
- Fibrin ball
  - Usually less than 1 cm in diameter
  - Adjacent to diaphragm
  - May change location on consecutive exams (loose within pleura)

Benign Pleural Mass

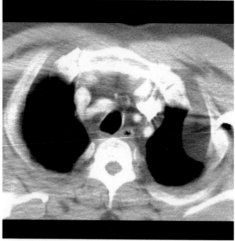

Pleural lipoma left apical hemithorax. Lipoma is the most common benign tumor of the pleural space. Lipomas may contain soft tissue strands but islands or nodules of soft tissue is more characteristic of a liposarcoma.

- Splenosis
  - Left sided
  - Associated with rib fractures from blunt chest trauma
  - Usually multiple
  - Most < 3 cm in diameter
  - Sharp, smooth contours

<u>CT Findings</u>
- Lipomas homogeneous fat density with fibrous strands
- Absent spleen in splenosis, other changes of trauma

<u>Nuclear Medicine Findings</u>
- Tc sulfur colloid uptake in splenosis

<u>Imaging Recommendations</u>
- Examination of choice to characterize pleural disease

Differential Diagnosis
<u>Liposarcoma</u>
- Fat minor component of soft-tissue mass
- Lipomas may have soft-tissue strands

<u>Fibrous Tumor of Pleura</u>
- May be associated with hypoglycemia or hypertrophic osteoarthropathy
- Large tumors inhomogeneous, often show contrast enhancement

<u>Mobile Pleural Masses</u>
- Lipoma
- Fibrin ball
- Foreign bodies
- Fibrous tumor of pleura

Pathology
<u>General</u>
- Malignant pleural masses more common than benign tumors

Benign Pleural Mass

- Etiology-pathogenesis
  - Splenosis requires laceration spleen and diaphragmatic tear following trauma, spleen fragments implant in pleural space, splenic tissue is functional, may develop in up to 15% with this injury
- Epidemiology
  - Lipoma most common benign pleural tumor

Gross Pathologic-Surgical Features
- Lipomas soft and moldable, predominantly fat
- Fibrin balls follow exudative effusions, common at autopsy but rarely seen radiographically
- Splenosis: Normal splenic tissue

Microscopic Features
- No specific features

Clinical Issues

Presentation
- Asymptomatic, incidentally discovered on chest radiographs

Treatment
- None, must be differentiated from more sinister process

Selected References
1. Müller NL: Imaging of the pleura. Radiology 186:297-309, 1993
2. Normand JP et al: Thoracic splenosis after blunt trauma: Frequency and imaging findings. AJR 161: 739-41,1993

Askin Tumor

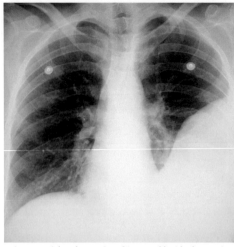

Askin tumor. Large peripheral mass in a 21-year old with chest pain. Margins are sharp and angle is obtuse with chest wall.

Key Facts
- Primitive neuroectodermal tumor (PNET)
- Most common pleural mass in young adults (especially women)
- Large unilateral pleural mass
- Widespread metastases lung, bone, sympathetic chain
- Prognosis poor (median survival 8 months)

Imaging Findings
Chest Radiograph
- Large, unilateral, pleural mass
- Rib and bone metastases
- Rapid growth
- Pleural effusion, smaller than mass
CT Findings
- Heterogeneous mass
- Pleural effusion > 90%
- Local extension into chest wall, mediastinum, and lung common
- Metastases to lung, bone, and mediastinal lymph nodes
- Unique metastases to sympathetic chain
MR Findings
- Heterogeneous mass, high signal intensity T1 and T2
- Enhance with gadolinium
Imaging Recommendations
- CT useful to characterize pleural masses and evaluate extent of disease

Differential Diagnosis
Lymphoma
- Pleural lymphoma usually a secondary manifestation of known disease
- Mass usually homogeneous without rib destruction
Ewings Sarcoma
- Centered on bone (rib), otherwise similar radiographic characteristics

Askin Tumor

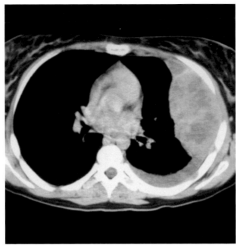

Askin tumor CT. Peripheral mass is inhomogeneous. No bone destruction. Small pleural effusion layering out posteriorly.

Rhabdomyosarcoma
- Identical radiographic characteristics, centered on chest wall with extension into lung

Neuroblastoma
- Involves sympathetic ganglion

Pathology
General
- Primitive neuroectodermal tumor (PNET)
- Genetics
  o Associated with translocation on chromosome 22
- Etiology-pathogenesis
  o May arise after radiation therapy for Hodgkin's disease

Gross Pathologic-Surgical Features
- Usually large, bulky tumors at diagnosis

Microscopic Features
- Small round cells ("blue"), similar to other PNET tumors
- Histology similar to Ewings tumor

Clinical Issues
Presentation
- Chest pain
- Most common pleural mass in young adults
- More common in females

Treatment
- Surgical excision
- Radiation therapy
- Chemotherapy

Askin Tumor

Prognosis
- Very poor, median survival 8 months

Selected References
1.   Winer-Muram HT et al: Primitive neuroectodermal tumors of the chest wall (Askin tumors): CT and MR findings. AJR 161:265-8, 1993
2.   Askin FB et al: Malignant small cell tumor of the thoracopulmonary region in childhood: A distinctive clinicopathologic entity of uncertain histogenesis. Cancer 43:2438-51, 1979

Pleural Metastases

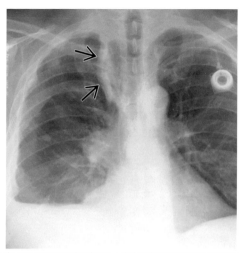

Metastatic adenocarcinoma to the pleura. Lobulated pleural thickening right hemithorax with extension into the azygos fissure (arrows). Small pleural effusion. The most common manifestation of pleural metastases is effusion.

Key Facts
- Pleura common metastatic site, especially from adenocarcinomas
- Most common finding pleural effusion
- Sensitivity pleural fluid cytology 60%
- Pleural masses or thickening uncommon on chest radiographs
- 20% asymptomatic
- Pleurodesis for symptomatic effusions

Imaging Findings
General Features
- Best imaging clue: Unexplained pleural effusion in patient with malignancy

Chest Radiograph
- Moderate-sized pleural effusion
  - In adults, 2nd most common cause pleural effusion (CHF #1)
  - Volume usually > 500 ml
- Multiple pleural masses, uncommon
- Diffuse pleural thickening

CT Findings
- May demonstrate anterior mediastinal mass in invasive thymoma
- Invasive thymoma may extend through diaphragmatic hiatus into abdomen or retroperitoneum
- Metastases may have variable enhancement
- May demonstrate mediastinal pleural involvement

Imaging Recommendations
- CT procedure of choice to evaluate pleural disease
- Useful for planning biopsy
- US useful for planning and directing thoracentesis

Pleural Metastases

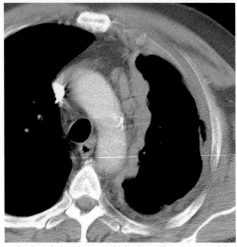

Metastatic renal cell. Lobulated pleural thickening with restriction of the hemithorax. Mesothelioma would be indistinguishable. However, malignant mesothelioma nearly always has a pleural effusion.

Differential Diagnosis
Mesothelioma
- Adenocarcinoma more common
- Pleural fluid 95% (vs. 50% for metastases)
- 10% have pleural plaques
- Nearly always symptomatic (metastases maybe asymptomatic)

Fibrothorax or Loculated Pleural Effusion
- Spares mediastinal pleura
- Pleural thickening not nodular
- Not circumferential in hemithorax
- May be calcified

Epithelioid Hemangioendothelioma
- Rare, old men

Pathology
General
- Sensitivity of pleural fluid cytology for metastases 60%
- Etiology-pathogenesis
  - Hematogenous, lymphatic, or direct spread to pleura
  - Adenocarcinoma most common tumor to metastasize to pleura
    - Lung cancer 40%
    - Breast 20%
    - Lymphoma 10%
    - Tumor of unknown origin 10%

Gross Pathologic-Surgical Features
- Pleural large extensive lymphatic network
- Metastases often flat, thin plaques, reason not seen on imaging studies
- Thymoma

Pleural Metastases

- o No pathologic features to separate invasive thymoma from benign thymoma, invasiveness dependent on imaging or surgical findings
- Lymphoma
  - o Usually secondary disease either recurrence or associated with other nodal disease
  - o Usually will not cause volume loss
  - o Will grow around ribs rather than destroying them

<u>Microscopic Features</u>
- Separation of mesothelioma from adenocarcinoma metastases difficult at light microscopy, requires special stains
- Epithelioid hemangioendothelioma vascular tumor with nests of tumor cells in myxoid stroma

Clinical Issues
<u>Presentation</u>
- May be asymptomatic (20%)
- Most common symptom dyspnea
- Nonspecific, dull, aching chest pain, anorexia, weight loss, malaise

<u>Treatment</u>
- Directed towards underlying malignancy
  - o Pleurodesis for symptomatic effusions
    - Tetracycline most common agent

<u>Prognosis</u>
- Generally signifies advanced incurable disease

Selected References
1. Muller NL: Imaging of the pleura. Radiology 186:297-309, 1993
2. Leung AN et al: CT in differential diagnosis of diffuse pleural disease. AJR 154:487-92, 1990

PocketRadiologist™
Chest
Top 100 Diagnoses

HYPERINFLATION & CYSTS

Emphysema

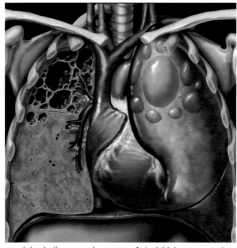

Bilateral upper lobe bullous emphysema. Apical blebs may rupture and cause spontaneous pneumothorax.

Key Facts
- Common medical problem, related to smoking
- Centriacinar most common, other types: Panlobular, paraseptal, irregular
- Chest radiography insensitive for mild disease
- Centriacinar predominately involves upper lung zones
- Panlobular predominately involves lower lung zones

Imaging Findings
Chest Radiograph
- Hyperinflation
  - Flat diaphragms
  - Widened retrosternal air space
  - Lung height increased
  - Small narrow heart
- Parenchymal areas of hypoattenuation
  - Inhomogeneous distribution
    - Arterial deficiency, increased branching angle of remaining vessels
  - Bullae
  - "Increased markings"
    - Not clearly understood, combination of bronchial wall thickening or superimposition emphysematous walls
- Secondary manifestations
  - Pulmonary arterial hypertension
    - Enlarged central pulmonary arteries and peripheral arterial pruning
- Sensitivity poor for early disease, rare false positives
  - Problem is recognition of loss of normal lung
  - Normal lung at chest radiography is 90% air, making detection of slight increases in air nearly impossible
- Crude correlation between indices of airways obstruction and radiographic findings

Emphysema

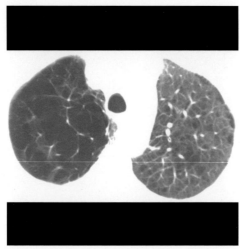

Severe centriacinar emphysema from long term smoking. Right upper lobe is nearly completely destroyed. Numerous discreet holes left upper lobe. Emphysema holes typically do not have a discernable wall. Emphysema is generally most severe in the upper lung zones.

HRCT Findings
- More sensitive than chest radiography
  - False negatives also occur with early disease
- Emphysematous holes usually have no discernable wall
- Central artery may remain visible surrounded by destroyed lung
- Objectively measured by assuming that lung with a threshold HU < -960 is emphysematous lung

Differential Diagnosis
Technical Considerations
- Low dose techniques may have false negatives
- Wide windows may cause false negatives

Asthma
- No parenchymal destruction, hyperinflation may be reversible

Constrictive Bronchiolitis Obliterans
- No parenchymal destruction, mosaic pattern

Athletic Hyperinflation
- Lung normal, young athlete

Pathology
General
- Abnormal enlargement of the airspaces distal to the terminal bronchioles accompanied by destructive changes of the alveolar walls without obvious fibrosis
- Etiology pathogenesis
  - Approximately 30% of the normal lung must be destroyed before pulmonary function deteriorates
  - Pulmonary function tests global summation of airways and lung
  - Emphysema usually inhomogeneous

Emphysema

- o Pulmonary function usually determined by structural integrity of lower lung zones
- o Patients may have anatomic emphysema without alteration of pulmonary function
- Centriacinar emphysema strongly associated with cigarette smoking
  - o Dose and time related
  - o Nearly all long term smokers will have anatomic emphysema

Gross Pathologic-Surgical Features
- Centriacinar
  - o Dilatation 2nd order respiratory bronchioles in secondary lobule
  - o Primarily involves upper lung zones
  - o Precursor may be respiratory bronchiolitis
- Panlobular
  - o Involves entire lobule
  - o Primarily involves lower lung zones
  - o Seen in senile emphysema and alpha-1-antiprotease deficiency
- Paraseptal
  - o Periphery of the secondary pulmonary lobule
- Irregular: Associated with scars
- Bullae
  - o Emphysema more than 1 cm in diameter with wall thickness < 1 mm

Clinical Issues

Presentation
- Dyspnea, shortness of breath
- Paraseptal emphysema at risk for spontaneous pneumothorax
- Pulmonary function (ATS criteria for functional emphysema)
  - o Obstruction
    - Increased total and residual volumes
    - Residue volume (RV) > 120% predicted
    - Decreased flow volumes
    - Forced expiratory volume one second (FEV_1) < 80% predicted
  - o Decreased diffusion capacity, < 80% predicted

Treatment
- Smoking cessation
  - o Pulmonary function will continue to decline
- Bronchodilators
- Vaccinations for pneumococcus
- Nutritional and physical therapy support
- Lung volume reduction surgery
  - o Undergoing randomized trial
  - o Candidates primarily those with inhomogeneous emphysema
- Bullectomy
  - o When bullae > 50% of hemithorax
  - o Lung otherwise normal as determined by CT
- Lung transplant for younger patients

Selected References
1. Thurlbeck WM et al: Emphysema: Definition, imaging, and quantification. AJR 163:1017-25, 1994
2. Stern EJ et al: CT of the lung in patients with pulmonary emphysema: Diagnosis, quantification, and correlation with pathologic and physiologic findings. AJR 162:791-8, 1994

Alpha 1-Antitrypsin Deficiency

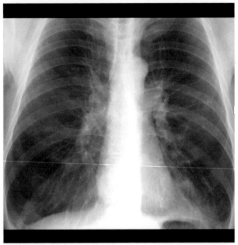

Alpha-1-antiprotease deficiency. Marked hyperinflation. Areas of arterial deficiency and hypoattenuation are most marked in the lower lobes with vascular redistribution to the upper lobes.

Key Facts
- Panlobular emphysema due to deficiency of alpha 1-antitrypsin
- Common Pi ZZ phenotype 1 in 2000
- Liver disease in infancy
- Emphysema develops prematurely, especially in smokers
- Predominantly involves lower lobes

Imaging Findings
Chest Radiograph
- Indirect signs of emphysema: Hyperinflation
  - Flat diaphragms
  - Widened retrosternal air space
  - Lung height increased
  - Small narrow heart
- Direct signs: Emphysema
  - Primarily involves lung base
  - Arterial deficiency and hypoattenuation
  - Bullae
  - "Increased markings"
    - Not clearly understood, combination of bronchial wall thickening or superimposition emphysematous walls
- Secondary manifestations
  - Pulmonary arterial hypertension
    - Enlarged central pulmonary arteries
    - Peripheral arterial pruning
CT Findings
- Not as easy to detect as centriacinar emphysema
- More sensitive than chest radiography
- Insensitive to mild disease
- Extensive areas of low attenuation

Alpha 1-Antitrypsin Deficiency

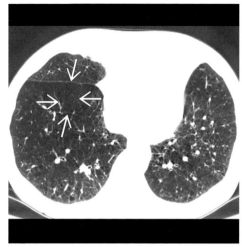

HRCT lung base. Mosaic perfusion. Ground glass represents more normal lung. Hyperinflated lobules (arrows) are nearly featureless with tiny arteries due to panlobular emphysema. Emphysema is inhomogeneous and does not destroy the lung uniformly.

- Reduction in size of pulmonary vessels
- Abnormal lung fades away, no normal lung to accentuate contrast differences
- Bullae common (33%)
- Bronchial wall thickening and bronchiectasis (40%)

Imaging Recommendations
- HRCT more sensitive than chest radiography

Differential Diagnosis

Lymphangiomyomatosis
- Women only, thin-walled cysts
- Chylous pleural effusion

Langerhans Cell Histiocytosis
- Predominantly upper lung zone
- Micronodules combined with bizarre shaped cysts

Neurofibromatosis
- Upper lobe bullae
- Basilar interstitial lung disease
- Neurofibromas, posterior mediastinal mass

Pathology

General
- Panlobular emphysema
- Genetics
  - Alpha-1-antiprotease blocks proteolytic enzymes
  - Coded by single gene chromosome 14
  - Single level determined by single allele derived from both parents
  - Normal phenotype (Pi MM)
  - Pi MZ have 60% normal levels no propensity for emphysema

Alpha 1-Antitrypsin Deficiency

- o Pi ZZ have 15% normal levels, need 35% to protect from emphysema
  - o Z variant single lysine for glutamic acid in M protein
- Etiology-pathogenesis
  - o Elastase-antielastase hypothesis
    - ▪ Natural elastases from neutrophils and macrophages normally neutralized by antiproteases
    - ▪ Imbalance causes emphysema
    - ▪ Animal model: Instillation of papain ("meat tenderizer") will induce emphysema
- Epidemiology
  - o Caucasians
  - o As common as cystic fibrosis, Pi ZZ 1 in 2000

Gross Pathologic-Surgical Features
- Emphysema predominantly involves the lower lung zones

Microscopic Features
- Panlobular: Uniformly involves the entire secondary pulmonary lobule, little or no fibrosis

Clinical Issues

Presentation
- Symptoms or signs rarely develop before age 55
- Smokers develop dyspnea age 40 compared to nonsmokers who become symptomatic at age 55
- Liver disease
  - o Homozygous deficiency in infancy
  - o Hepatosplenomegaly, may lead to cirrhosis
  - o Hepatoma second most common cause of death

Treatment
- Smoking cessation
- Augmentation therapy with IV alpha-1-protease inhibitor
- Gene therapy in future

Prognosis
- Life expectancy decreased even in nonsmokers

Selected References
1. Spouge D et al: Panacinar emphysema: CT and pathologic findings. J Comput Assist Tomogr 17:710-3, 1993
2. Guest PJ et al: High resolution computed tomography (HRCT) in emphysema associated with alpha-1-antitrypsin deficiency. Clin Radiol 45:260-6, 1992

Lymphangiomyomatosis (LAM)

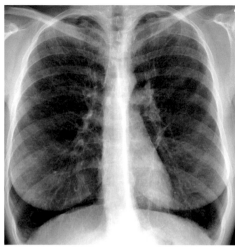

LAM. Lungs are markedly hyperinflated in this young woman. Scattered, coarse, interstitial thickening throughout the lung. Combination of interstitial thickening and hyperinflation should suggest LAM.

Key Facts
- Women of child-bearing age
- Chest radiography: Paradoxical reticular interstitial disease with increased lung volumes
- CT: Numerous thin-walled cysts with intervening normal lung
- Often present with spontaneous pneumothorax
- Most eventually develop pleural or pericardial chylous effusion
- Associated findings include mediastinal and retroperitoneal adenopathy
- Renal angiomyolipoma (15%)

Imaging Findings
General Features
- Best imaging clue: Coarse interstitial thickening in hyperinflated lungs

Chest Radiograph
- Reticular interstitial thickening, (coarse honeycombing)
- Normal or enlarged lung volume
  - Paradoxical observation as Interstitial Lung Disease (ILD) is restrictive and decreases lung volumes
- Small to moderate pleural effusions
- Spontaneous pneumothorax (40%)

CT/HRCT Findings
- Reticular thickening on chest radiograph represents superimposed cysts
- Thin-walled cysts uniform in size, increase in size and number as disease progresses
- Cysts will eventually completely replace lung
- Diffuse distribution, no predilection for any region of the lung
- Intervening lung normal
- CT may demonstrate cysts when chest radiograph and PFTs normal
- Pleural or pericardial effusion (chylous, 60%)
- Mediastinal and retroperitoneal adenopathy

Lymphangiomyomatosis (LAM)

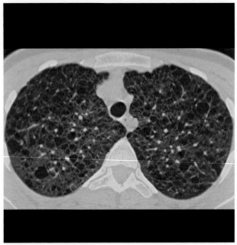

HRCT. *Numerous thin-walled cysts are uniformly distributed throughout the lung. Lung between cysts is normal. Diagnosis: LAM.*

- Renal angiomyolipoma (15%)
- Scattered ground-glass opacities (may represent hemorrhage)

Imaging Recommendations
- HRCT diagnostic findings, more sensitive than chest radiography

Differential Diagnosis

Langerhans Cell Histiocytosis
- Young smokers, centrilobular micronodules, bizarre-shaped cysts
- No pleural effusion

Emphysema
- Older, holes have no definable wall
- No pleural effusion

Neurofibromatosis
- Holes predominately upper lung zones, basilar interstitial lung disease

Pathology

General
- Hamartomatous proliferation of smooth muscle around lymphatics, airways, and blood vessels
- Genetics
  - Identical pathologic findings found in 1-2% of patients with tuberous sclerosis (women only)
  - Nonfamilial (tuberous sclerosis, however, autosomal dominant)
- Etiology-pathogenesis
  - Predilection for premenopausal women suggests estrogen plays a role in pathogenesis
- Epidemiology
  - Women of child-bearing age

Gross Pathologic-Surgical Features
- Cysts uniformly distributed throughout the lung
- Chylous effusion

Lymphangiomyomatosis (LAM)

- Enlarged thoracic duct and lymph nodes with hamartomatous smooth muscle proliferation

Microscopic Features
- Normal tissue disorganized, no specific microscopic features

Clinical Issues

Presentation
- Presenting symptoms: Dyspnea and pneumothorax
- Hemoptysis 30%
- Pulmonary function tests
  - Obstructive indices with hyperinflation
  - Decrease carbon monoxide diffusion in the lung (DLCO)

Treatment
- Discourage air travel
  - Increases risk of pneumothorax
- Pregnancy counseling
  - Pregnancy may exacerbate disease
- Progesterone and oophorectomy
  - Variable success
- Lung transplant
  - Disease may recur in transplanted lung
- Pleurodesis for effusions or pneumothorax may worsen pulmonary function

Prognosis
- Survival 50% five years
  - Death due to respiratory failure, occasionally renal failure

Selected References
1. Sullivan EJ: Lymphangioleiomyomatosis: A review. Chest 114:1689-703, 1998
2. Muller NL et al: Pulmonary lymphangiomyomatosis: Correlation with radiographic and functional findings. Radiology 175:335-9, 1990

Laryngotracheal Papillomatosis

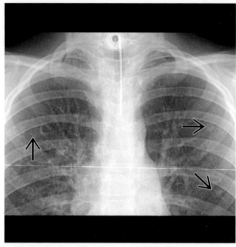

Child with laryngotracheal papillomatosis. Multiple ill-defined pulmonary nodules (arrows). Tracheostomy for laryngeal squamous cell carcinoma.

Key Facts
- Laryngeal nodules due to human papilloma virus, usually self-limited infection
- < 1% seed the lung
- Multiple solid or cystic pulmonary nodules
- Nodules very slow growth
- Predominant dorsal distribution at CT (gravity seeding)
- At risk to develop squamous cell carcinoma (2%)

Imaging Findings
Chest Radiograph
- Multiple solid or cavitated nodules
  - As nodules enlarge more likely to cavitate
- Thick or thin wall
- Slow growth (years)
- Air-fluid level suggests superinfection
- Atelectasis curiously rare
- Tracheal wall thickening or nodularity

CT Findings
- Dorsal distribution, may be related to gravity and dependent seeding of the lung
- Useful to evaluate trachea and airways for papillomas
- Useful to evaluate change in nodules for bronchogenic carcinoma
- Nodules communicate with adjacent airways

Differential Diagnosis
Metastases
- Variable size sharply defined
- Cavitation usually seen in squamous cell histology or sarcomas

Laryngotracheal Papillomatosis

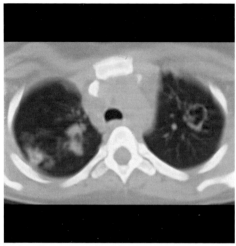

Laryngotracheal papillomatosis. Both solid and cavitated nodules. Typically, nodules are more profuse in the dorsal lung.

Wegener's
- Subglottic stenosis
- Paranasal sinus or renal disease

Pneumatoceles
- Transient and usually follow known insult (trauma, infection, hydrocarbon ingestion)
- Trachea normal

Lymphangiomyomatosis
- Women, cysts randomly distributed
- Chylous pleural effusion
- Trachea normal

Langerhans Cell Histiocytosis
- Nodules and/or cysts, primarily in upper lung zones
- Trachea normal

Emphysema
- Holes have no wall
- Older with smoking history
- Trachea normal

Sjögren's
- History of sicca syndrome
- 1/3 have thin-walled cysts
- Trachea normal

Pathology
General
- Etiology-pathogenesis
  - Laryngeal infection with human papilloma virus, usually self-limited
  - < 1% seed the lung
  - Airway dissemination
    - Surgical manipulation of laryngeal papillomas increases risk of dissemination

Laryngotracheal Papillomatosis

o Lung seeding usually apparent in children or young adults

Gross Pathologic-Surgical Features
• Sessile or papillary lesions with vascular core covered by squamous epithelium

Microscopic Features
• Lung and laryngeal lesions composed of squamous cells, cavities lined with squamous epithelium

Clinical Issues

Presentation
• Symptoms: Dyspnea, hemoptysis, obstructive pneumonia depend on size, number, and position of papillomas

Natural History
• Lung nodules grow very slowly, usually measured in decades
• 2% incidence of squamous cell carcinoma degeneration
  o Any change in nodule should be investigated for malignant transformation

Treatment
• Usually self-limited infection
• Laser ablation of laryngeal or airway lesion

Prognosis
• Disseminated disease: death due to respiratory failure
• Secondary bronchogenic carcinoma

Selected References
1. Kawanami T et al: Juvenile laryngeal papillomatosis with pulmonary parenchymal spread. Case report and review of the literature. Pediatr Radiol 15:102-4, 1985
2. Kramer SS et al: Pulmonary manifestations of juvenile laryngotracheal papillomatosis. AJR 144:687-94, 1985

PocketRadiologist™
Chest
Top 100 Diagnoses

HEART & PERICARDIAL

Cardiac Size and Contour

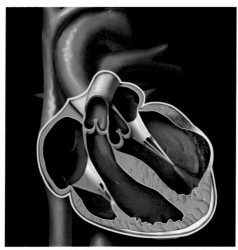

Left ventricular aneurysm. Thinning of the anterolateral wall of the left ventricle is usually the result of a remote myocardial infarction. This focal convexity often shows dystrophic calcification and akinesis. Aneurysms may manifest clinically as congestive heart failure, arrhythmias or systemic emboli.

Key Facts
- Subjective size estimate more accurate than objective measurements
- Normal-sized heart does not rule out heart disease
- Doubling myocardial wall thickness may not enlarge cardiac size
- CT and MRI excellent modalities to evaluate individual chambers, wall thickness and volumes

Imaging Findings
Chest Radiograph
- Subjective size estimate, however, more accurate than any objective measurements
  - Sensitivity 50% compared to angiographically determined left ventricular volume
  - Normal cardiothoracic ratio < 0.45
- Cardiac size determined by
  - Chamber volumes
    - Radiographic diameter between systole and diastole
    - 50% < 0.3 cm
    - 95% < 1 cm
    - 5% 1–1.7 cm
  - Myocardial thickness
    - Contributes little to overall size, doubling wall thickness still within range of normal for change between diastole and systole
    - 80% of radiographic heart size determined by chamber volumes
  - Pericardial volume
    - Normal fluid volume 25 to 50 ml
- Cardiomegaly
  - Conditions with volume overload lead to larger cardiac dimensions than conditions due to pressure overload
  - Heart size from regurgitation exceeds that due to stenosis

Cardiac Size and Contour

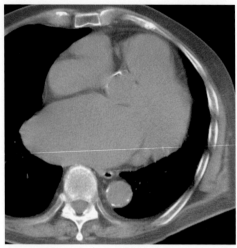

Left atrial enlargement from mitral regurgitation. Left atrium is markedly enlarged out of proportion to the other cardiac chambers. Chambers are larger in regurgitation compared to stenosis.

- Left atrium enlargement
  - Right-sided retrocardiac double density
  - Enlarged left atrial appendage (3rd mogul)
  - Carinal angle widening
  - Oblique line from edge of double density to middle of the left main stem bronchus should be < 7 cm normally
  - Lateral radiograph: Posterior displacement left upper lobe bronchus
- Left ventricle enlargement: Apex shifted down and out
- Right ventricle enlargement: Apex uplifted and shifted sideways (boot shape)
  - Lateral radiograph: Anterior encroachment anterior clear space
- Right atrium enlargement
  - Ice-cream shaped right heart border
- Small heart
  - Spurious: With hyperinflation small size due to widening of thorax and elongation of pericardium which is tethered to the flat diaphragms
- True (microcardia)
  - Addison's disease
  - Concentration camp starvation (myocardium last muscle to be used for nutrition)
  - Tension pneumopericardium
- Focal bulge
  - Pericardial defects
    - Prominent air-filled notch between aorta and pulmonary artery
    - Air interposed between heart and diaphragm inferiorly
    - Heart shifted to the left
  - True aneurysm: Typical location anterolateral or apical wall
  - False aneurysm: Typical location posterolateral and diaphragmatic wall

Cardiac Size and Contour

CT Findings
- More accurate and sensitive method to characterize and quantitate cardiac size

MR Findings
- Most accurate method to determine volume, cardiac output, ejection fraction and regurgitant volumes

Differential Diagnosis

Spurious Cardiomegaly
- Full expiration: High diaphragms decreases thoracic width
- Supine position: Short AP tube film distance and poor inspiration

Pericardial Effusion
- Widening epicardial stripes
- Water bottle-shaped heart

Mediastinal Lipomatosis
- Diffuse fat at CT

Thymolipoma
- Thymic mass composed of fat and soft tissue draped over heart

Pathology

Gross Pathologic-Surgical Features
- Left ventricle normal dimensions
  - Normal end diastolic volume: 70 ± 20 ml/mm^2
  - Normal end systolic volume: 25 ± 10 ml/mm^2 (ejection fraction 0.67)
  - Normal wall thickness 11 ± 2 mm
  - Cavity diameter
    - Systole 33.6 ± 3.8 mm
    - Diastole 46.4 ± 5.5 mm
- Right atrium maximum volume 77 ± 11 ml/mm^2
- Left atrium maximum volume 55 ± 5 ml/mm^2
- Right ventricle normal dimensions
  - Normal end diastolic volume: 70 ± 15 ml/mm^2
  - Normal end systolic volume: 40 ± 10 ml/mm^2 (ejection fraction 0.6)
  - Normal wall thickness < 3 mm

Clinical Issues

Presentation
- Heart disease with normal-sized heart
  - Aortic stenosis: Dilatation seen with failure and critical stenosis
    - Enlarged ascending aorta (post-stenotic dilatation)
  - Systemic hypertension
  - Mitral stenosis
  - Acute myocardial infarction
  - Hypertrophic cardiomyopathy
  - Restrictive cardiomyopathy
  - Constrictive pericarditis

Selected References
1. Rose CP et al: The limited utility of the plain chest film in the assessment of left ventricular structure and function. Invest Radiol 17:139-44, 1982
2. Edwards WD et al: Standardized nomenclature and anatomic basis for regional tomographic analysis of the heart. Mayo Clin Proc 56:479-97, 1982

Cardiac Calcification

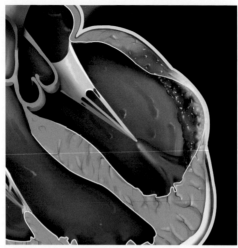

Calcified left ventricular aneurysm. Infarcted myocardium may eventually calcify.

Key Facts
- Valvular calcification usually associated with stenosis
- Direct relationship between coronary artery calcification and stenosis
- CT may be useful to screen for coronary artery calcification
- Mitral annulus calcification a benign degenerative process
- 10% of atrial myxomas calcify

Imaging Findings
Chest Radiograph
- General
  - Myocardial calcification generally linear or arcuate
  - Valve calcification generally nodular or clumped
  - Quantity of calcification directly related to degree of stenosis
- Aortic and Mitral valves
  - PA: Valves overlap adjacent to spine, difficult to separate; clues
    - Aortic valve: In profile, horizontally positioned
    - Mitral valve: En face, vertically positioned
  - Lateral view: Heart is football shaped, "lace" of the football
    - Aortic valve is anterior, mitral valve is posterior to laces
  - Aortic valve calcification
    - Vertical club shape, because raphe in bicuspid valve first to calcify
- Mitral annulus
  - Large C or horseshoe-shaped calcification
  - Measures 10 cm in circumference
- Left atrium
  - Diffuse in severe rheumatic mitral stenosis
  - Focal wall calcification usually located posterior wall left atrium due to jet effect from mitral regurgitation (MacCallum's patch)
- Coronary artery

Cardiac Calcification

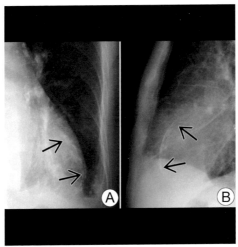

Left ventricular aneurysm. (A, B) Thin linear calcification overlying anterior cardiac apex (arrows). True aneurysm usually from large infarct. Infarct is old as it takes years to calcify.

- o Cardiac triangle: Vertical border – medial border spine, superior diagonal border – left heart border, inferior border – approximately 1/3 the distance from the left bronchus to diaphragm at the level of the "shoulder" of the left ventricle
  - ▪ Visible calcification highly associated with significant stenosis
- Atrial myxomas
  - o 10% calcify, mulberry type similar to fibroids
  - o Myxomas may have flat border (due to origin from interatrial septum)

CT Findings
- More sensitive than chest radiography to detect calcium
- Valve calcification may be incidental without hemodynamic stenosis
- Mitral valve prolapse may be secondary to the abnormal shape of chest wall with cardiac entrapment
  - o Narrowed AP diameter, large area of contact anterior myocardium with chest wall, figure-of-8 cross-sectional shape thorax
- Coronary artery calcification
  - o Frequent finding in otherwise healthy adults, signifies atherosclerosis
  - o Greater the quantity the greater the likelihood of significant stenosis (not necessarily related to the site of the calcium)
  - o Absence of calcification does not rule out unstable plaque
    - ▪ Consistent with a lowered risk for near term cardiovascular event
  - o Measured with electron beam CT or multispiral CT
    - ▪ Calcium score derived by computer calculating the area and density of each coronary artery calcification (above a certain threshold, typically 130 HU)
    - ▪ Calcium score compared to gender and age matched populations

Differential Diagnosis
Pericardial Calcification vs. Myocardial
- Usually right sided (left sided)

Cardiac Calcification

- Diffuse and extensive (focal)
- Spares left atrium and apex (spares AV groove)
- Lateral view: Over pulmonary outflow tract (under pulmonary valve)

Pathology
General
- Calcification usually dystrophic due to abnormal tissue or flow hemodynamics, may be degenerative
- Etiology-pathogenesis
  o Mitral annulus calcification a degenerative process
  o Infarcts: Usually seen in large infarcts, requires years to develop (>6)
  o Valve calcification uncommon in mitral valve prolapse or in tricuspid or pulmonic valve pathology
- Epidemiology
  o Mitral annulus calcification more common in elderly women, incidence increased in patients with Idiopathic Hypertrophic Subaortic Stenosis (IHSS)
  o Bicuspid aortic valve 2% of population
  o Myxomas, 50% all cardiac tumors (left atrium 75%, right atrium 25%)
Gross Pathologic-Surgical Features
- Bicuspid aortic valves, 90% calcified
  o True or (false in parenthesis) left ventricle aneurysms
    ▪ Wide neck (narrow neck)
    ▪ LAD disease (RAD disease)
    ▪ Typical location anterolateral or apical wall (posterolateral or diaphragmatic wall)
Microscopic Features
- Calcification part of the intimal plaque in atherosclerosis

Clinical Issues
Presentation
- Calcified infarct at increased risk for sudden death
- Coronary artery calcification screening with CT may be useful for those with atypical chest pain or to evaluate those with strong family history of coronary artery disease or other risk factors for coronary artery disease
- True aneurysm clot rarely embolizes
- True aneurysm may serve as arrhythmogenic source or result in CHF
- False aneurysm is true perforation, may rupture result in sudden death
Treatment
- Surgical replacement abnormal valves, bypass procedures for coronary artery disease
- Lifestyle modifications for coronary artery disease
- Resect aneurysms for CHF, embolic disease, or intractable arrythmia
Prognosis
- Left atrial calcification may complicate valve replacement due to risk of bleeding and embolization

Selected References
1. Lee VS et al: Atypical and unusual calcifications of the heart and great vessels: Imaging findings. AJR 163:1349-55, 1994
2. Freundlich IM et al: Calcification of the heart and great vessels. CRC Crit Rev Clin Radiol Nucl Med 6:171-216, 1975

Pericardial Effusion

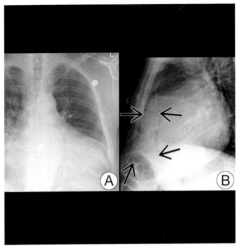

Pericardial effusion. (A) Massive cardiomegaly with a water bottle configuration. (B) Pericardial stripe on the lateral view is widened (arrows).

Key Facts
- Numerous infectious, immunologic, neoplastic, or traumatic causes
- Normal fluid 25 ml to 50 ml
- Chest radiograph: Water bottle shape, widened epicardial stripe
- CT recesses may be confused with enlarged nodes or aortic dissection

Imaging Findings
Chest Radiograph
- Cardiomegaly
  - Water bottle configuration
    - Gravity layering of fluid inferiorly in pericardial sac
- Widened epicardial stripe lateral view
  - Normal epicardial stripe
    - < 2 mm thick
    - Normally seen in 70% normal chest radiographs
    - Pericardium sandwiched between mediastinal fat and epicardial fat
- Widened subcarinal angle
  - Normal 40–70 degrees
- Left pleural effusion
- Tamponade
  - Enlarged heart
  - Pulmonary edema rare
  - Widened superior mediastinum due to dilatation of superior vena cava

CT Findings
- Evaluates entire pericardial space
- Recesses common adjacent to major vessels
  - Retroaortic recess normally seen in 95%
  - Superior aortic recess seen in 90%
  - Left pulmonic vein recess seen in 60%

Pericardial Effusion

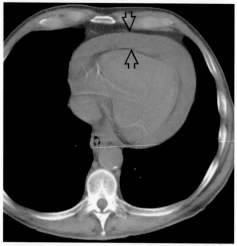

CT large pericardial effusion. Heart tends to settle posteriorly in the pericardial sac so that the majority of fluid accumulates anteriorly. Separation of the epicardial fat from the anterior mediastinal fat (arrows) accounts for the pericardial stripe on the lateral examination.

- Tamponade findings
  - Pericardial effusion
  - Atrial dilatation
  - SVC and IVC dilatation
  - Pleural effusions
  - Ascites
  - Dilatation hepatic veins
  - Elongation ventricles

MR Findings
- More sensitive than CT for fluid

Echocardiography
- Unable to evaluate entire pericardium
- Primary modality to evaluate all cardiac diseases

Differential Diagnosis
Cardiac Chamber Enlargement
- Normal epicardial stripe

Thymolipoma
- Enlarged soft tumor conforms to cardiac shape, easily separated from heart at CT

Mediastinal Adenopathy
- Pericardial recesses at CT may be confused for enlarged lymph nodes or aortic dissection
- Retroaortic recess blends into ascending aorta, enlarged node separate from edge of aorta

Differentiation
- CT, MRI or echocardiography useful to separate pericardial from other causes of enlarged cardiac silhouette

Pericardial Effusion

Pathology
General
- Etiology-pathogenesis of pericardial effusion
  - Pericardial sac will hold 150–250 ml of fluid before acutely tamponade
  - Slow accumulations may exceed 3 L without tamponade
  - Pericardial disease often associated with left pleural effusion
  - Hydrostatic
    - Pulmonary hypertension
    - CHF
    - Uremia
    - Hypoalbuminemia
  - Infections
    - Viral, bacterial and fungal and TB
  - Immunologic
    - Systemic lupus erythematosus
    - Rheumatoid arthritis
    - Postpericardiotomy syndrome (including Dressler's – post MI)
    - Periarteritis nodosa
    - Rheumatic fever
  - Drugs
    - Procainamide
    - Hydralazine
    - Coumadin
  - Metastases
    - Lung, breast, lymphoma
  - Trauma: Iatrogenic hemorrhage
    - Post cardiac cath or surgery
  - Idiopathic
    - Hypothyroidism, usually massive pericardial effusion
    - Radiation therapy

Gross Pathologic-Surgical Features
- Normal pericardium surrounds heart and attaches to ascending aorta
- Normal pericardial fluid 25 ml to 50 ml

Clinical Issues
Presentation
- Tamponade
  - Dyspnea, dilated neck veins
- Postpericardiotomy syndrome (including Dresslers – post MI)
  - 2-4 weeks following event
  - Fever, chest pain
  - Autoimmune hypersensitivity reaction
  - Usually self-limited
  - May treat with steroids

Treatment
- Pericardiocentesis for sampling and acute drainage for tamponade

Selected References
1. Breen JF: Imaging of the pericardium. J Thorac Imaging 16:47-54, 2001
2. Kremens V: Demonstration of the pericardial shadow on the routine chest roentgenogram: A new roentgen finding. Radiology 64:72-80, 1955

Pericardium, Calcium & Masses

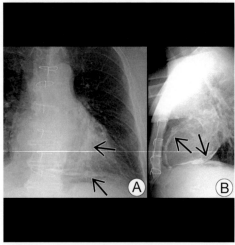

Pericardial calcification. (A) Coarse linear calcification (arrows) best seen on the lateral view (B).

Key Facts
- Most patients with pericardial calcification will have constrictive pericarditis
- Pericardial cysts common benign disorder
- Fat pad sign following mantle radiation therapy signifies lymphoma in inadequately treated diaphragmatic lymph nodes
- Absence of pericardium: Heart shifts to the left and surrounded by air

Imaging Findings
<u>Chest Radiograph</u>
- Calcification
  - Eggshell calcification predominantly inferior and right sided
  - With constrictive pericarditis
    - Widened superior mediastinum
    - Lack of pulmonary edema
    - Elevated diaphragms due to ascites
- Cysts
  - Partly spherical with sharp smooth contours
  - Usually located right cardiophrenic angle
  - 2 to 30 cm in diameter
- Absence of left pericardium
  - "Snoopy dog" appearance
    - Heart shifted to left (Snoopy's nose)
    - Air interposed between aortic arch and main pulmonary artery
    - Prominent left atrial appendage (Snoopy's ear)
    - Air interposed between left hemidiaphragm and inferior heart border
- Neoplastic
  - Metastases usually cause effusion, not masses
  - Primary tumors rare
    - Sarcomas, large bulky tumors

Pericardium, Calcium & Masses

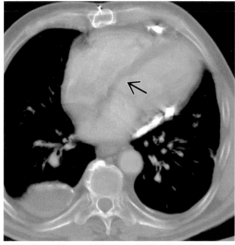

Pericardial calcification. The ventricles are slightly elongated. Angulation of the interventricular septum (arrow) suggests the development of constrictive pericarditis. Previous pericardial stripping for constrictive pericarditis. Now has recurrent symptoms.

CT Findings
- Constrictive pericarditis findings
  - Calcification
  - Pericardial effusion
  - Atrial dilatation
  - SVC and IVC dilatation
  - Pleural effusions
  - Ascites
  - Dilatation hepatic veins
  - Elongation ventricles

MR Findings
- Similar to CT
- Calcification not as well identified

Imaging Recommendations
- Echocardiography primary tool to investigate pericardium
- CT and MRI useful to examine entire pericardium
- CT and MRI useful to distinguish myocardial from pericardial disease
- CT and MRI useful to further characterize pericardial masses

Differential Diagnosis

Myocardial Calcification
- Pericardial
  - Usually right sided (less cardiac motion)
  - Diffuse and extensive
  - Spare left atrium and apex
  - AV groove
  - Lateral view: Over pulmonary outflow tract
- Myocardial
  - Usually left sided

Pericardium, Calcium & Masses

- o Focal
- o Apex typical location
- o Spares AV groove
- o Lateral view: Projects under pulmonary valve

Pericardial Epicardial Fat Pad
- Fat density at CT

Morgagni Hernia
- Bowel or mesenteric fat in anterior hernia sac

Enlarged Pericardial Lymph Nodes
- "Fat pad" sign
- Cardiac blockers often used with mantle therapy to prevent premature arteriosclerosis
- Pericardial and diaphragmatic lymph nodes inadequately treated
- Recurrence may be manifested by enlarging "fat pads"

Thymic Cysts or Thymolipoma
- Cysts will have fluid density at CT or MRI, thymolipomas contain fat, thymus usually separate from pericardium

Loculated Pleural Effusion
- Fluid density at CT, usually can be separated from uninvolved pericardium

Lung Mass
- Separate from pericardium at CT, bronchogenic carcinoma can directly extend into pericardium

Pathology
General
- Etiology-pathogenesis
  - o Cysts and partial absence developmental anomalies
  - o Constrictive pericarditis
    - Viral origin
    - Tuberculosis
    - Rheumatic
    - Idiopathic

Gross Pathologic-Surgical Features
- > 50% with pericardial calcification will have constrictive pericarditis
- < 90% with constrictive pericarditis will have pericardial calcification

Clinical Issues
Presentation
- Usually asymptomatic incidental finding
- Constrictive pericarditis
  - o Dyspnea, shortness of breath

Treatment
- Surgical stripping pericardium, difficult to remove entire pericardium
- May recur

Selected References
1. Breen JF: Imaging of the pericardium. J Thorac Imaging 16:47-54, 2001
2. Rozenshtein A et al: Plain-film diagnosis of pericardial disease Semin Roentgenol 34:195-204, 1999

Pacemaker & Defibrillator Leads

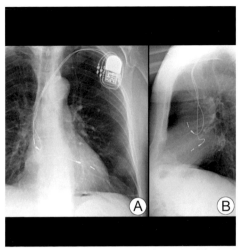

Pacemaker tip malpositioned in left ventricle. On the PA view (A), the tip is high and does not extend to the left apex. The lateral (B) is crucial. The tip does not project past the posterior half of the heart.

Key Facts
- Transvenous pacemakers common
- Complications, malposition, lead fracture, and perforation easily overlooked
- Lead positioned in coronary sinus should be suspected on frontal radiograph if tip directed to left shoulder
- Coronary sinus or cardiac vein position definitively determined by posterior position on lateral radiographs

Imaging Findings
<u>Chest Radiograph (Transvenous Pacemakers)</u>
- Normal position
  - Ideal position, pacer lead tip at apex of right ventricle (cardiac apex on PA view)
  - Lateral view, tip should be positioned anteriorly, directed at sternum
  - For sick sinus syndrome or arrhythmia detection, a lead may be deliberately positioned in the coronary sinus or middle cardiac vein
- Abnormal position
  - Coronary sinus
    - Lead course very similar to ideal position on PA view
    - Clue: on PA view, tip will be directed to left shoulder
    - Lateral view: tip will be posterior along the border of the heart
  - Lead fracture
    - Common locations: Attachment to generator, 1st rib – clavicular crossing ("osseous pinch"), and ventricular tip
    - Some pacemaker models have nonopaque segments close to the generator where dual connectors bifurcate
  - Dislodgement
    - Widely changing position of tip on serial radiographs

Pacemaker & Defibrillator Leads

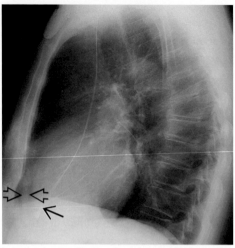

Perforation by pacemaker tip. The tip extends to epicardial fat (arrow). In addition there is a small pericardial effusion (open arrows).

- Normally there may be some alteration of position due to changes between systole and diastole
- Pacemaker twiddling: patient may fiddle with generator and wind up the electrodes much like retrieving a fishing line
  o Myocardial perforation
    - Suspect when tip is within 3 mm of the epicardial fat or edge of the heart
  o Infection
    - Most common location is generator pocket
    - May extend down the pacemaker leads
    - Soft tissue swelling or fluid collection at generator site

Chest Radiograph (Implantable Cardioverter Defibrillators)
- Typically 2 electrodes, one SVC (defibrillator) and apex right ventricle (defibrillating and sensing)
- Leads are larger and have a coiled spring appearance as compared to pacemaker leads
- Complications similar to transvenous pacemakers
- Relief loop in the left subclavian region often constructed to help prevent lead migration
- Normally, there may be a lucency just distal to proximal electrode not to be confused with a fracture
- Implantable defibrillators (anterior and posterior cardiac patches) less common
- Patches often crinkle with time normally due to fibrosis
- Crinkling may also be due to infection with fluid accumulation beneath the patch

CT Findings
- May be useful to examine implanted defibrillator patches for fluid accumulation

MR Findings
- MR contraindicated in patients with pacemakers or defibrillators

Pacemaker & Defibrillator Leads

- Magnetic field may generate electrical currents in the pacemaker leads

Other Modality Findings
- Fluoroscopy may be useful to examine leads for incomplete fracture or dislodgement
- Rarely done by radiologists

Imaging Recommendations
- Chest radiographs usually sufficient for diagnosis
- Fluoroscopy may be useful to examine dynamic position of leads, rarely done

Differential Diagnosis
- None

Pathology

General
- Epidemiology
  - Incidence of radiographic abnormalities may approach 20%
    - Malposition 5%
    - Lead fracture 2%
    - Perforation 5%
    - Infection 5%

Gross Pathologic-Surgical Features
- Right ventricular wall normally only 4-5 mm thick and is easily perforated

Clinical Issues

Presentation
- Transvenous pacemakers common for treatment of various arrhythmias
- Implantable cardioverter defibrillators used to treat ventricular tachycardias
- Malfunction may produce syncope, perforation may cause twitching of abdominal muscles or hiccupping from diaphragm stimulation

Treatment
- Replacement fractured wires
- Perforation treated by withdrawing wire and rescrewing into myocardium

Selected References
1. Daly BD et al: Nonthoracotomy lead implantable cardioverter defibrillators: Normal radiographic appearance. AJR 161:749-52, 1993
2. Steiner RM et al: The radiology of cardiac pacemakers. Radiographics 6: 373-99, 1986

PocketRadiologist™
Chest
Top 100 Diagnoses

PULMONARY ARTERY

Pulmonary Embolism

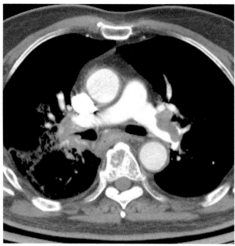

CT pulmonary angiography. Bilateral central pulmonary emboli. Left saddle embolus. Patchy consolidation right lung may be early infarct. Right hilum also enlarged from bronchogenic carcinoma.

Key Facts
- Common disease, any hospitalized patient at risk
- Chest radiograph nonspecific, 10% normal
- Pulmonary infarcts uncommon, may be any shape or size
- CT angiography examination of choice, highly sensitive and specific
- Outcomes for negative CT angiograms good (< 1% embolic rate)
- Pulmonary angiography and V/Q scanning rarely performed

Imaging Findings
Chest Radiograph
- 10% normal
- Most abnormalities nonspecific
- Vascular alteration
  - Focal enlargement central pulmonary artery (knuckle sign)
    - Commonly right interlobar pulmonary artery
    - Due to physical presence of clot
  - Focal oligemia (Westermark sign)
    - Due to vascular obstruction
- Pulmonary infarct
  - < 10% embolic episodes result in infarction
  - Infarction more common in those with underlying cardiopulmonary disease
  - May develop immediately or delayed 2-3 days following embolus
  - Any size or shape
    - Usually peripheral or in lower lung zones
    - Often associated with small pleural effusion
  - Evolution
    - Initially ill-defined, over time become sharply defined
  - Resolution
    - 50% clear completely usually within 3 weeks

Pulmonary Embolism

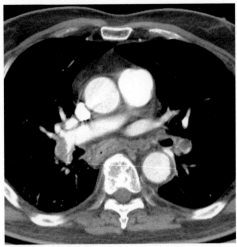

CT pulmonary angiogram. Emboli extend into lobar pulmonary arteries. CT is less sensitive for subsegmental emboli.

- ▪ Others leave linear scars (Fleischner lines)
  - o Hampton's hump
    - ▪ Peripheral wedge-shaped opacity with rounded apex pointing toward the hilum
  - o Infarcts "melt"
    - ▪ Maintain their initial shape and shrink over time
    - ▪ Pneumonia and edema generally "fade" away

V/Q Scanning Findings
- Indirect indicator of clot, does not directly visualize the clot
- High sensitivity but poor specificity
  - o Normal perfusion scan excludes embolus
- Interobserver agreement poor for low and indeterminate V/Q category (30%)

CT Findings
- Spiral or electron beam CT revolutionized diagnosis of PE
- Directly visualizes clot in central pulmonary artery
- High sensitivity and specificity (> 90%)
- Pitfalls
  - o Poor bolus
  - o Hilar lymph nodes
  - o Breathing artifacts
  - o May miss subsegmental emboli
  - o Oblique arteries may require oblique reconstructions to adequately visualize
- High observer agreement
- Can be combined with scanning pelvis and thighs for thromboembolic disease
- Outcomes of negative CT angiograms good
  - o DVT or PE 0.5%
  - o Fatal embolism 0 to 0.7%

Pulmonary Embolism

Pulmonary Angiography Findings
- Rarely performed in clinical practice
- Considered gold standard
  - 25% false negative for small subsegmental emboli
- Interobserver agreement poor for subsegmental emboli (>30%)

Differential Diagnosis
Pneumonia
- Common in critically ill, nonspecific opacities must consider embolus
Atelectasis
- Common in critically ill, nonspecific opacities must consider embolus

Pathology
General
- Pulmonary emboli end result of thrombosis in peripheral veins generally of the lower extremities
- Epidemiology
  - Considered 3rd most common cause of death
  - Any hospitalized patient at risk for emboli, other risk factors
    - Trauma
    - Surgery
    - Obesity
    - Pregnancy
    - Malignancy
    - MI
    - Antithrombin-III deficiency
Gross Pathologic-Surgical Features
- Hemodynamic consequences
  - > 50% reduction vascular bed leads to pulmonary hypertension and right heart failure
- Deep venous clot fragments in right heart, an average of 8 vessels embolized

Clinical Issues
Presentation
- No telltale signs, symptoms, or laboratory studies that strongly suggest PE
Treatment
- Anticoagulation and fibrinolysis
  - Hemorrhage complications in 2 – 15%
- IVC filter if contraindications to drug therapy
Prognosis
- Good with appropriate therapy, must maintain high index of suspicion as mortality untreated disease 20%
- Outcomes for untreated subsegmental emboli unknown
  - Outcome following negative pulmonary angiograms or CT good

Selected References
1. Elliott CG et al: Chest radiographs in acute pulmonary embolism. Results from the International Cooperative Pulmonary Embolism Registry. Chest 118:33-8, 2000
2. Remy-Jardin M et al: Spiral CT angiography of the pulmonary circulation. Radiology 212:615-36, 1999

Pulmonary Hypertension

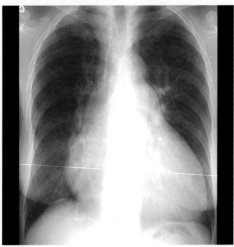

Primary pulmonary hypertension. Massive cardiomegaly. Main pulmonary artery is enlarged.

Key Facts
- Classified as pre or post capillary
- Primary pulmonary hypertension affects predominantly young women
- COPD most common secondary cause of hypertension
- Enlarged central pulmonary arteries with rapid tapering, right ventricular (RV) hypertrophy
- Septal thickening, centrilobular nodules, pleural and pericardial effusions and mediastinal adenopathy suggest post-capillary hypertension

Imaging Findings
Chest Radiograph
- Enlarged central pulmonary arteries
- Rapid pruning peripheral pulmonary arteries
- Cardiomegaly with right ventricular hypertrophy
- Associated findings with secondary disease
  - COPD: Hyperinflation, emphysema, bullae, bronchiectasis
  - Interstitial lung disease: End-stage honeycombing
- Normal transverse diameter of right interlobar pulmonary artery
  - < 16 mm men
  - < 14 mm women
  - Sensitivity for mild hypertension = 50%
  - Sensitivity for severe hypertension = 75%
- Edema, septal thickening and small pleural effusions more common with post-capillary pulmonary hypertension

CT Findings
- Normal transverse diameter of main pulmonary artery < 28.6 mm
- Useful to exclude chronic pulmonary embolism as cause of hypertension
- Better demonstrates right ventricular hypertrophy
- Central ground-glass opacities, septal thickening, pleural effusions, pericardial effusions and mediastinal adenopathy suggest post-capillary pulmonary hypertension

Pulmonary Hypertension

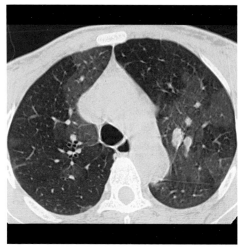

Pulmonary artery hypertension. Mosaic perfusion. Hypoattenuating areas have small arteries. Arteries are larger in ground glass areas. No air-trapping at expiration (not shown).

- Centrilobular nodules may also represent cholesterol granulomas which are seen in up to 25% of patients with pulmonary hypertension
- Mosaic attenuation pattern common in pulmonary hypertension
  - Geographic ground-glass attenuation represents normal or hyperperfused lung
  - No air trapping with expiratory CT
  - Vessels in hypoattenuated lung have decreased caliber due to either vascular obstruction or hypoxic vasoconstriction
- Intimal calcification with longstanding, severe hypertension
- Peripheral lobular or wedge-shaped opacities in those who develop pulmonary infarcts

MR Findings
- Similar to CT

Ventilation Perfusion Scan Findings
- Usually low probability scans except in patients with chronic thromboemboli which has a high probability pattern

Differential Diagnosis
Adenopathy
- Hilum more lobulated may have abnormal mediastinal contours from adenopathy

Pathology
General
- Hemodynamic vascular changes due to elevated pressure from either pre or post capillary obstruction
- Etiology-pathogenesis
  - Pre-capillary
    - Congenital left to right shunts, chronic thromboemboli

Pulmonary Hypertension

- Metastases especially hepatoma, gastric carcinoma, renal cell, right atrial sarcoma, breast
- Schistosomiasis, AIDS
- IV drug abuse: Talcosis, portal hypertension (2%)
- Primary pulmonary hypertension
- End-stage honeycombing, COPD, sleep apnea
  - o Post-capillary
    - Veno-occlusive disease, mediastinal fibrosis
    - Mitral stenosis; LV dysfunction
    - Obstruction left atrial mass (myxoma)
- Epidemiology
  - o Primary pulmonary hypertension: women 3rd decade
  - o 1% with acute pulmonary emboli will go on to chronic disease
  - o Pulmonary veno-occlusive disease, 1/3rd children
    - Idiopathic or associated with pregnancy, bone marrow transplantation, drug toxicity

Gross Surgical-Pathologic Features
- Normal resting mean pulmonary artery pressure < 20 mm Hg
- Intimal hyperplasia
- Smooth muscle hypertrophy
- Chronic emboli may have webs and bands and recanalized clots
- Right ventricular hypertrophy

Microscopic Features
- Necrotizing arteritis and capillary plexiform lesion in primary pulmonary hypertension
- Capillary hemangiomatosis in pulmonary veno-occlusive disease
- Centrilobular cholesterol granulomas in 25%

Clinical Issues

Presentation
- Nonspecific symptoms: Dyspnea, easy fatigue, chest pain
- Pulmonary veno-occlusive disease often preceded by flu-like illness

Treatment
- Oxygen
- Anticoagulation for thromboemboli
  - o Consider IVC filter
  - o Thromboendarterectomy
- Prostaglandin I_2 (epoprostenol) for primary hypertension
  - o Vasodilator given by continuous IV infusion
  - o Side effects: Jaw pain, erythema, diarrhea, arthralgias
  - o May cause death in those with post-capillary hypertension
- Lung with or without heart transplant

Prognosis
- Poor

Selected References
1. Frazier AA et al: From the archives of the AFIP: Pulmonary vasculature: Hypertension and infarction. Radiographics 20:491-524; quiz 530-491, 532, 2000
2. Sherrick AD et al: Mosaic pattern of lung attenuation on CT scans: Frequency among patients with pulmonary artery hypertension of different causes. AJR 169:79-82, 1997

PocketRadiologist™
Chest
Top 100 Diagnoses

AORTA

Aortic Aneurysm

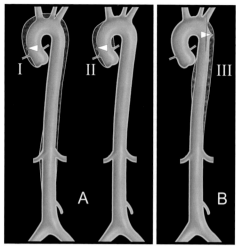

Type A aortic dissection (DeBakey types I and II) involves the ascending aorta and requires surgical repair. Type B (DeBakey type III) involves the descending aorta and is treated medically.

Key Facts
- Aneurysm should be considered in differential for any mediastinal mass
- Saccular aneurysm > 6.5 cm significant risk for rupture
- Chest radiography may be normal in patient with dissection
- Dissecting aneurysms of ascending aorta usually surgically repaired

Imaging Findings
<u>Chest Radiograph</u>
- Normal ascending aorta < 4 cm in diameter
- Normal descending aorta < 3 cm in diameter
- Normal aging: Loss of elasticity elongates aorta. Because aorta fixed, the aorta buckles with a tortuous course
- Any mediastinal mass should be considered as a vascular aneurysm, a needle or scalpel could find a surprise
- Curvilinear calcification clue to vascular origin
- Saccular aneurysm > 6.5 cm significant risk for rupture
- Dissection
  - Wide mediastinum or widening aortic arch
  - Displaced intimal calcification from aortic wall > 10 mm (5%)
  - Mediastinal mass effect, tracheal shift, depression left main bronchus
  - Left pleural effusion
  - Sensitivity 80% (chest may be normal), specificity 80%
- Calcification ascending aorta
  - Typical atherosclerotic plaque uncommon
  - Syphilis or Type II hyperlipidemia
- Ascending aorta aneurysm
  - Dissection
  - Annuloaortic ectasia (Marfan's, Ehlers-Danlos)
  - Syphilis or aortitis

Aortic Aneurysm

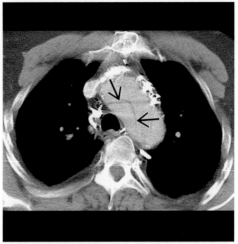

Marfan's with aortic dissection. Intimal flap (arrows) is evident in the aortic arch. Both the true and false lumen are patent. Involvement of the ascending aorta is a key feature that must be evaluated.

- Aortic arch aneurysm
  - Traumatic pseudoaneurysm, ductus aneurysm
  - Mycotic, coarcatation, dissection
- Descending aorta aneurysm
  - Dissection, penetrating ulcer, atherosclerosis

CT Findings
- Procedure of choice to demonstrate aneurysm and vascular anatomy
- Dissection
  - Utility to separate Type A (ascending aorta) dissection (requires surgery) from Type B (descending aorta) (treated medically)
  - Goal visualize true and false lumens separated by flap
  - Which is true and which is false lumen?
    - Connect true lumen with undissected portion on sequential images
  - False lumen
    - Beak sign: Acute angle between the dissected flap and the outer wall, angle may contain thrombus
    - Cobwebs: Thin strands crossing lumen
    - Intraluminal thrombus; entire lumen may be thrombosed
    - Largest lumen usually the false lumen
- Dissection pitfalls
  - False negatives: Poor contrast enhancement
  - False positives: Streak artifacts
- Penetrating ulcer
  - Mid-descending aorta, may be multiple
  - Wall hematoma acutely high density, best seen in noncontrast CT

MR Findings
- Does not require intravenous contrast but not as accurate as CT
- Can be used to evaluate for aortic valvular regurgitation
- More sensitive to detect hematoma in penetrating ulcer

Aortic Aneurysm

- Useful for serial surveillance of those at risk, e.g. Marfan's syndrome

Transesophageal Echocardiograph
- Can be done at bedside, operator dependent
- Less accurate: ascending aorta obscured by air-filled trachea

Differential Diagnosis

Tortuosity (Aging) of the Aorta
- No displacement intimal calcification, not dilated

Mediastinal Teratoma
- May spontaneously bleed with sudden change in size

Achalasia
- Air-fluid level, absent gastric air bubble

Pathology

General
- True aneurysm composed of all layers of aortic wall, false aneurysm represents a perforation of wall
- Etiology-Pathogenesis
  o Greatest hydraulic stress right lateral wall ascending aorta or descending aorta in proximity of ligamentum arteriosum
  o Predisposing conditions aneurysm: Atherosclerosis, trauma, mycotic, cystic medial necrosis
  o Aortitis: Syphilis (now rare), giant cell aortitis, ankylosing spondylitis, RA, rheumatic fever, relapsing polychondritis, Reiter's, Behcet disease, Takayasu
  o Predisposing factors dissection: Cystic medial necrosis, hypertension, penetrating ulcer, bicuspid aortic valve, relapsing polychondritis
- Epidemiology
  o Penetrating ulcers: Hypertensive elderly men

Gross Pathologic-Surgical Features
- Intimal tear spirals with false lumen lies anterior and right in the ascending aorta and posterior and left in the descending aorta

Microscopic Features
- None

Clinical Issues

Presentation
- Asymptomatic to sudden death
- Aortic dissection may be painless (15%)

Treatment
- Ascending (Type A) surgical
  o Graft used to close false lumen
  o May rupture into pericardium (tamponade)
  o Compress coronary artery
  o Aortic regurgitation (50%) may require valve replacement
- Descending (Type B) medical antihypertensive drugs

Prognosis
- Dissection: 25% die in first 24 hours

Selected References
1.   LePage MA et al: Aortic dissection: CT features that distinguish true lumen from false lumen. AJR 177:207-11, 2001
2.   Posniak HV et al: CT of Thoracic aortic aneurysms. Radiographics 10:839-55, 1990

Aortic Anomalies

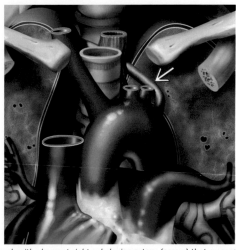

Left aortic arch with aberrant right subclavian artery (arrow) that crosses to the right side posterior to the esophagus.

Key Facts
- All mediastinal masses should be considered vascular until proven otherwise
- Aberrant right subclavian artery most common aortic anomaly
- Aberrant artery origin usually dilated (diverticulum of Kommerell) and may rarely cause dysphagia (dysphagia lusoria)
- Right aortic arch with mirror imaging branching usually associated with congenital heart disease
- "Figure 3" sign classic radiographic abnormality in coarctation of aorta
- Pseudocoarctation morphologically similar but no pressure gradient across stenosis and no collateral vessels to cause rib notching

Imaging Findings
Chest Radiograph
- Aberrant right subclavian artery
  - Mass effect posterior to trachea in Raider's triangle
    - Clear space posterior to trachea, anterior to vertebral bodies, and superior to aortic arch
  - Oblique posterior impression in esophagram pointing to right shoulder
- Right aortic arch
  - Right paratracheal mass
  - Aberrant left subclavian artery
    - Diverticulum of Kommerell may look like the normal left aortic arch
- Coarctation (pseudocoarctation)
  - "Figure 3" sign
    - Indentation at coarctation
    - Lower bulge post-stenotic dilatation descending aorta
    - Proximal bulge ascending aorta
  - Inferior rib notching

Aortic Anomalies

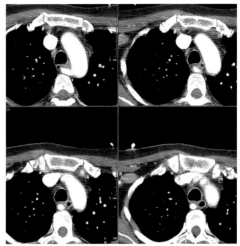

Aberrant right subclavian artery is a common anomaly. The subclavian artery passes behind the esophagus and trachea. Occasionally the origin (diverticulum of Kommerell) is dilated and may cause dysphagia (dysphagia lusoria).

- Enlarged tortuous intercostal arteries that serve as collateral vessels
- Notching not seen before 6 years of age
- Unilateral if aberrant subclavian artery
  - Retrosternal undulating tubular opacity
    - Subclavian artery collateral to internal mammary artery
  - Pseudocoarctation same as coarctation but without pressure gradient across stenosis
    - No collateral flow, no rib notching

CT Findings
- Aberrant right subclavian artery
  - Origin distal to left subclavian artery
  - Courses posterior to trachea and esophagus
- Right aortic arch
  - Aberrant left subclavian artery
    - Courses posterior to trachea and esophagus
  - Mirror imaging branching usually associated with congenital heart disease
- Coarctation
  - Axial less than ideal to image isthmus
  - CT evaluation requires helical scanning with reconstructions in oblique, sagittal, or coronal planes

MR Findings
- Advantages
  - No radiation
  - Multiplanar capabilities
  - Valvular morphology and function
  - Intracardiac morphology

Aortic Anomalies

Differential Diagnosis
Mediastinal Mass Any Compartment
- All mediastinal masses should be considered vascular until proven otherwise especially if
  - Adjacent to known vascular structures
  - Mural calcification
  - Oval or round shape with smooth contour
  - Poor visualization in orthogonal view

Pathology
General
- Anomalies common anatomic variants
- Genetics
  - Aberrant right subclavian artery: Incomplete regression of the primitive distal right aortic arch
- Right aortic arch: Interruption of embryologic double arch between the left common carotid artery and the left subclavian artery

Gross Pathologic-Surgical Features
- Coarctation: Obstructing membrane at the level of aortic isthmus

Clinical Issues
Presentation
- Aberrant right subclavian artery
  - 1.5% most common anomaly of the aortic arch
  - Enlarged diverticulum of Kommerell may cause dysphagia (dysphagia lusoria)
  - 1/3 of Down syndrome patients with congenital heart disease have aberrant right subclavian artery
- Right aortic arch
  - Mirror imaging branching
  - Associated with congenital heart disease
    - Tetralogy of Fallot
    - Ventricular septal defect
    - Truncus arteriosus
  - Aberrant left subclavian artery
    - Not associated with congenital heart disease
- Coarctation
  - Upper extremity hypertension
  - Associated lesions
    - Bicuspid aortic valve (25%)
    - Aneurysms at coarctation or circle of Willis
    - PDA or VSD
    - Turner syndrome

Treatment
- None for anomalies unless symptomatic
- Surgery or balloon angioplasty for short segment stenosis

Prognosis
- Morbidity and mortality of surgical repair

Selected References
1. Proto AV et al: Aberrant right subclavian artery: Further observations. AJR 148:253-7, 1987
2. Salomonowitz E et al: The three types of aortic diverticula. AJR 142:673-9, 1984

PocketRadiologist™
Chest
Top 100 Diagnoses

TRAUMA

Aortic Transection

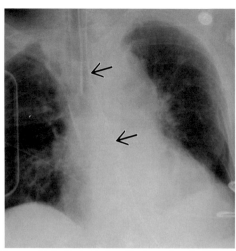

Blunt chest trauma. Mediastinal widening with obscuration of aortic arch. NG tube is deviated to the right (arrows). Left main bronchus is depressed inferiorly. Chest radiograph is sensitive but not specific. Angiography or CT required.

Key Facts
- 15% of mortalities in MVA, 95% occur at aortic isthmus
- Chest radiograph sensitive but nonspecific
- Signs of transection may be absent
- Angiography rapidly being replaced by CT angiography
- CT angiograms directly visualize tear
- False-positive conventional and CT angiograms from atherosclerotic plaques and normal ductus diverticulum

Imaging Findings
Chest Radiograph
- Will not visualize the tear, indirect signs only from hemorrhage
- Signs of transection sensitive but not specific
  - Widening superior mediastinum
  - Abnormal contour aortic arch, obscuration of AP window
  - Tracheal shift to the right
  - NG shift to the right
  - Widening paraspinal stripe
  - Depressed left mainstem bronchus
  - Left apical cap
  - 1st rib fracture (protected by clavicle and scapula, requires considerable force to break, direct indicator of severity of trauma and thus likelihood of aortic transection)
- Any of the above signs require further investigation to rule out transection
- Signs centered at aortic arch, the most common location for transection
- Normal chest radiograph previously considered rare
  - CT angiography has shown injures in up to 15% of those with no signs of aortic transection on radiographs (false negative chest radiograph)
- Chronic aneurysm (2% survivors)

Aortic Transection

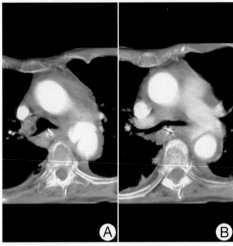

CT angiography. Sequential CT images. Proximal descending aorta has abnormal contour (A) with small pseudosacculation. NG tube is deviated (B). Mediastinal fat is completely effaced by blood.

   o Calcified mass aorticopulmonary window

<u>CT Findings</u>
- Initially used to reduce false-positive chest radiographs by demonstrating other causes of mediastinal widening
- CT angiography directly demonstrates aortic tear, markedly reducing the need for aortography
- Signs
  - o Periaortic hematoma
  - o Pseudo diverticulum or irregular contour aortic wall
  - o Intimal flap
- Requires intravenous contrast and helical scanning
- Accuracy: Sensitivity 100%, specificity 80%
- False positives: Motion or streak artifact, plaque, ductus diverticulum, adjacent bronchial artery

<u>Aortography Findings</u>
- Considered gold standard for evaluating aorta and great vessels
- False negatives and false positives low (see below)
- Using chest radiograph as guide, perform 10 negative angiograms for each tear
- Small risk of rupture
- Rapidly being replaced by CT angiography
- False positives
  - o Ductus diverticulum 25%
    - Smooth, gently sloping shoulders
    - Tears have irregular margins and steep shoulders
  - o Ulcerated plaque
    - More common in older patients, other plaques in aorta
  - o Aortic spindle (15%)
    - Congenital narrowing at ligamentum arteriosum
  - o Infundibulum of the bronchial-intercostal trunk

Aortic Transection

- False negatives, once considered rare
  - CT angiography has shown a 5% miss rate for aortic injury

MR Findings
- Limited in transporting and monitoring critically injured patients

Transesophageal Echocardiography Findings
- Will demonstrate intimal tears and transection
- More difficult to do in severely injured patients
- Limited availability

Differential Diagnosis
Widened Mediastinum
- In acute trauma, false positives due to rotation (especially to patient's right), supine positioning, expiration

Pathology
General
- Etiology pathogenesis
  - Deceleration hypothesis: Aorta fixed at ligamentum arteriosum
  - Osseous pinch: Manubrium and first ribs rotate and impact spine causing shear injury
- Epidemiology
  - Accounts for 15% fatalities in MVA

Gross Pathologic-Surgical Features
- 95% at aortic isthmus
  - From origin left subclavian artery to ligamentum arteriosum
- Other 5% ascending aorta or descending aorta at diaphragmatic hiatus
- Ascending aorta 20% coroner's results, rarely survive to reach hospital
- Transverse circumferential tear: Intima and media tear with intact adventitia (60%)
- Noncircumferential tears more common posteriorly

Clinical Issues
Presentation
- Urgent diagnosis, 50% expire 24 hours if untreated
- Majority have no signs or symptoms, nonspecific chest pain, dyspnea
  - Acute coarctation syndrome rare
    - Upper extremity hypertension
    - Decreased femoral pulses
- Multiple associated injuries
  - Diaphragm rupture, lung contusion, rib fractures, head injury

Treatment
- Surgical repair (also recommended for chronic aneurysms)
- Beta-adrenergic blocking agents to decrease wall stress
- Endovascular stent grafts promising

Prognosis
- 85% survival, paraplegia 10% (directly related to cross-clamp time)

Selected References
1. Dyer DS et al: Can chest CT be used to exclude aortic injury? Radiology 213:195-202, 1999
2. Patel NH et al: Imaging of acute thoracic aortic injury due to blunt trauma: A review. Radiology 209:335-48, 1998

Diaphragmatic Rupture

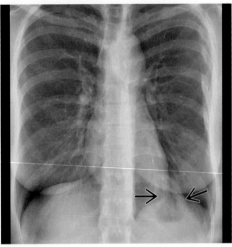

Remote history of blunt chest trauma. Stomach has hour-glass configuration as it crosses the ruptured diaphragm (arrows). Contour abnormality AP window proved to be chronic aortic pseudoaneurysm. Multiple healed left rib fractures.

Key Facts
- Prevalence: 5% in blunt trauma patients
- Delayed diagnosis common
- Chest radiography usually abnormal
- Specific signs: Air-filled viscus in hemithorax
- Additional signs CT: Dependent viscera sign
- New pleural effusion in patient with hernia heralds the onset of strangulation

Imaging Findings
Chest Radiograph
- Abnormal 90% but diagnostic in only 50%
- Air-filled bowel in hemithorax
- Tip of NG tube in hemithorax
  - Tear usually spares esophageal hiatus
  - NG tube will course normally into abdomen and then traverse into hemithorax if stomach herniated
- Elevated diaphragm > 7 cm
- Diaphragmatic contour changes shape with change in position
- Abnormal diaphragmatic contour
- Contralateral mediastinal shift
- Strangulation
  - Pleural effusion in patient with hernia should suggest strangulation
  - With open communication, pleural fluid should not accumulate
  - Omental fat may simulate pleural effusion, including layering on decubitus examination
CT Findings
- Dependent viscera sign
  - Liver or bowel in contact with posterior ribs

Diaphragmatic Rupture

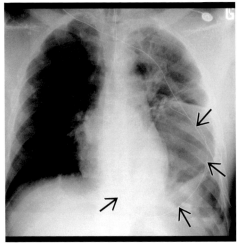

Blunt chest trauma. Herniated stomach through diaphragmatic rent. NG tube courses through esophageal hiatus then into stomach (arrows).

- Visceral herniation with focal constriction of bowel or liver (collar sign)
- Discontinuity of the crus of the diaphragm
- Left diaphragmatic tear: Sensitivity 80%, specificity 100%
- Right diaphragmatic tear: Sensitivity 50%, specificity 100%
- Reformats in coronal and sagittal plane important for right-sided injury

MR Findings
- Similar to CT, more difficult to perform in acute setting

Barium Gastrointestinal Findings
- Longstanding method to demonstrate herniation
- Approximation and narrowing of afferent and efferent bowel loops (pinched limbs) through the diaphragmatic defect (collar sign or kissing birds sign)

Other Findings
- US and liver-spleen scans have all been used to diagnose diaphragmatic tears

Differential Diagnosis
Eventration of Diaphragm
- Bowel loops will not be approximated in eventration

Diaphragm Paralysis
- Paradoxical motion at fluoroscopy

Enlarged Liver
- No collar sign for liver

Loculated Pleural Effusion
- No bowel, crus intact

Paraesophageal Hernia
- Tear rare at esophageal hiatus

Subphrenic Abscess
- Diaphragm intact, separate from bowel

Diaphragmatic Rupture

Pathology
General
- Spontaneous healing uncommon, herniated abdominal contents prevent approximation of edges of tear
- Epidemiology
  - Prevalence 5% blunt chest trauma

Gross Pathologic-Surgical Features
- Radial tear extending from central tendon posterolaterally
- > 2 cm long, most more than 10 cm long
- Left sided 70%, right cushioned by liver
- CT diaphragmatic defects 5%
  - Normal process of aging
  - More common in women

Clinical Issues
Presentation
- Acute
  - Multiple associated injuries
    - Rib fractures 40%
    - Pelvic fractures 50%
    - Liver or spleen laceration
    - Aortic tear 5%
    - Head injury
  - Diagnosis delayed 25%
  - Intubated patient on positive pressure may prevent herniation
  - Herniation may be obscured by other injuries
- Latent
  - Asymptomatic or mild epigastric discomfort
  - Spontaneous respiration (negative intrapleural pressure)
    - Gradient for progressive herniation of abdominal contents
    - High index of suspicion important throughout the hospital course of trauma patients
- Obstructive
  - Strangulation of bowel
    - 85% strangulation within 3 years; however, cases have been undiagnosed for decades
    - Morbidity and mortality strangulation 30%
  - Obstructive symptoms, fever, chest pain

Treatment
- Surgical correction

Prognosis
- Excellent
- Morbidity and mortality higher with strangulation

Selected References
1. Killeen KL et al: Helical CT of diaphragmatic rupture caused by blunt trauma. AJR 173:1611-6, 1999
2. Fataar S et al: Diagnosis of diaphragmatic tears. Br J Radiol 52:375-81, 1979

Blunt Chest Trauma

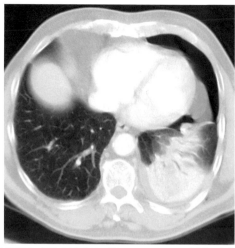

Blunt chest trauma, lung contusion. Homogeneous consolidation left lower lobe. Large pneumothorax. Contusion is a "black and blue mark" in the lung.

Key Facts
- Pulmonary contusions and lacerations appear soon after trauma
- Radiography usually shows patchy or homogeneous airspace opacities
- Pneumatoceles and hematomas indicate pulmonary laceration
- CT - best to show small lacerations or hemopneumothorax
- Lacerations are slow to resolve, several weeks to months
- May occur without thoracic bony injury

Imaging Findings
Chest Radiograph
- Opacities appear soon after trauma, < 6 hours
- Adjacent to ribs and vertebral bodies
- Located at impaction or contrecoup lung injury
- Irregular patchy areas of airspace consolidation (mild)
- Perihilar increased interstitial markings
  - Hemorrhage and edema in peribronchovascular interstitium
- Diffuse extensive homogeneous consolidation (severe)
- Improvement within 24 to 48 hours
- Complete clearing within 10 days
  - Except when develop ARDS/respiratory failure
- Lacerations
  - May appear hours or days after trauma
  - At point of maximum impact or contrecoup location
  - Thin-walled air-filled cysts (pneumatoceles)
    - With or without air-fluid levels
    - May fill with blood (hematoma) rarely hematomas expand
    - Single or multiple
    - Oval or spherical
    - Unilocular, multilocular
    - 2 to 14 cm diameter

Blunt Chest Trauma

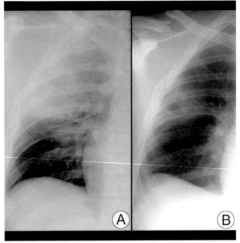

Large contusion right upper lobe (A) has nearly completed resolved over a 3 day period (B). Multiple rib fractures and right clavicular fracture.

- Persist for up to 4 months
- Gradual decrease in size, 1-2 cm/week
- Weeks to months to resolve

CT Findings
- More sensitive than radiography
- 1-2 mm of subpleural lung spared
- May see small lacerations with air-fluid levels
- Hematoma
  o Slight increased attenuation centrally
  o Enhancing rim
  o May be confused with nodule
- Hemopneumothorax, especially from Type 3 injury (see Pathology section)

Imaging Recommendation
- Chest radiographs usually sufficient to follow course of blunt trauma

Differential Diagnosis

Aspiration
- Identical radiographic findings
- Aspiration common in head trauma

Pneumonia
- Identical radiographic findings, occurs later in hospital course
- If contusion worsens after 48 hours, consider superinfection

Pathology

General
- Contusions very common with blunt chest trauma
- Etiology pathogenesis
  o Sudden deceleration tearing capillaries and small blood vessels
  o Direct impaction or impalement (fractured rib)

Blunt Chest Trauma

Gross Pathologic-Surgical Features
• Air spaces filled with blood
Staging
• Type 1: From blunt trauma and sudden compression of pliable chest
• Type 2: Lung compressed and lacerated between chest wall and vertebra
• Type 3: Punctured lung by fractured rib
• Type 4: Pleural adhesions tear at lung when chest wall compressed

Clinical Issues
Presentation
• Usually no specific symptoms from contusions, pneumatoceles, or hematomas
Treatment
• Supportive therapy, surveillance for other major organ injuries, observe for complications
• Complications: Infection, hemopneumothorax, or hemoptysis
Prognosis
• Variable, usually related to other injures like aortic transection

Selected References
1.   Mirvis SE et al: Imaging in acute thoracic trauma. Semin Roentgenol 27:184-210, 1992

Chest Wall Trauma

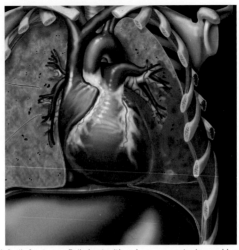

Multiple left rib fractures, flail chest with pulmonary contusion and hemorrhage.

Key Facts
- Rib fractures common, 1st rib fracture marker for severity of trauma
- Flail segments impair ventilation
- Thoracic spine fractures may have similar signs to aortic transection
- Most thoracic spine fractures result in neurologic injury
- Most common location thoracic spine injury thoracolumbar junction

Imaging Findings
<u>Chest Radiograph</u>
- Thoracic Spine
  - Pedicle thinning with a slight increase in the interpediculate distance at the level of thinning normally seen at the thoracolumbar junction in 7%
  - Rule of 2's: 2 mm is the normal upper limits for difference in
    - Interspinous or interlaminar distance
    - Interpedicular distance (transverse and vertical)
    - Anterolisthesis or retrolisthesis with flexion and extension
    - Facet joint width
    - Height of anterior and posterior vertebral bodies
  - Bone integrity
    - Anterior height < posterior height
    - Ratio 0.80 males, 0.87 females
    - Spinous process midline projecting slightly below anterior endplate
    - Double spinous processes clue to spinous process fracture
  - Instability if one of the following
    - Displaced vertebra
    - Widened interlaminar or interspinous distance
    - Perched or dislocated facet joints
    - Increased interpediculate distance
    - Disrupted posterior vertebral body line
  - Posttraumatic collapse (Kommell's disease)
    - After minor trauma

Chest Wall Trauma

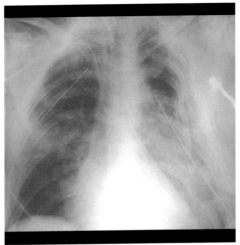

Blunt chest trauma, bilateral contusions and chest tube drainage. Left flail chest. Note: The costal hook sign for ribs 3-8 indicative of a large flail segment.

- Avascular necrosis vertebral body
- Associated with intravertebral or intradiskal vacuum disc
- Sternum
  - Direct trauma: Posterior displacement lower sternal fragment
  - Indirect trauma: Posterior displacement upper sternal fragment
    - Spinal flexion "buckles" the sternum
- Ribs
  - 30% sensitivity (normal to miss rib fractures)
  - Ribs 4 through 9 most commonly fractured
  - Fractures usually multiple
  - Common following blunt chest trauma
  - 1st rib fracture
    - Marker for severity of chest trauma
    - Protected by clavicle, scapula
    - 2% have bronchial tear and 10% have aortic transection
  - Flail chest (up to 20% of patients with major trauma)
    - 2 or more adjacent ribs with segmental fractures (more than 2 fractures or more than 5 adjacent rib fractures)
    - Costal hook sign: Elephant trunk shaped ribs (rotation of segmental fractures)

<u>CT Findings</u>
- Primarily used to investigate skeletal integrity

<u>MR Findings</u>
- Primarily used to investigate spinal cord, disc, and ligaments
- Optimal timing for cord imaging: 24-72 hours following injury
- Cord hemorrhage associated with poor prognosis for neurologic recovery
- Cord edema associated with better prognosis for neurologic recovery

Chest Wall Trauma

Differential Diagnosis
Aortic Transection
- 50% of patients with spinal cord fracture will have signs of aortic transection
  - Mediastinal widening 50%
  - Apical cap 50%
  - Thickened right paratracheal stripe 60%

Pathology
General
- Etiology-pathogenesis
  - Thoracic spine flexion
    - Results in compression fractures (50% of all fractures)
  - Axial compression
    - Results in burst fracture (15% of all fractures)
  - Hyperflexion
    - Results in flexion-distraction (seat belt) fracture (15% of all fractures)
  - Shearing results in fracture-dislocation (5% of all fractures)
  - Flail chest
    - Pendelluft breathing, paradoxical motion flail segment with ventilation (in with inspiration, out with expiration)
- Epidemiology
  - Thoracic spine fractures, 15% have multiple levels
  - <5% have both aortic transection and cord injury

Gross Pathologic-Surgical Features
- Spinal canal smallest in thoracic spine
  - Limited leeway for fragments to cause cord injury
- Facets
  - Normally facets in thoracic spine in coronal plane (facets face in)
  - Facets in lumbar spine in oblique sagittal plane (facets face out)
  - Transition zone between thoracic and lumbar facet orientation (T_{9-11}) most common location for fracture with flexion injuries

Clinical Issues
Presentation
- Thoracic spine 90% have cord injury
  - Thoracolumbar junction fractures more common to injure cord than upper thoracic spine fractures
- Rib fractures usually of little consequence
  - External splinting by rib corset may result in hypoventilation and pneumonia
- Flail chest
  - May not be clinically evident in 1/3
  - Large segment may result in respiratory impairment

Treatment
- Surgical fixation thoracic spine fractures
- Positive pressure ventilation flail segment until chest wall stabilizes

Selected References
1. el-Khoury GY et al. Trauma to the upper thoracic spine: Anatomy, biomechanics, and unique imaging features. AJR 160:95-102, 1993
2. DeLuca SA et al. Radiographic evaluation of rib fractures. AJR 138:91-2, 1982

Tracheobronchial Rupture

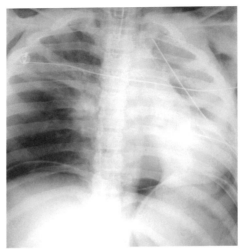

MVA. Subcutaneous emphysema left chest wall and mediastinal air (continuous diaphragm sign). Bilateral pneumothoraces and pneumoperitoneum. Collapse left lower lobe. Air collections were progressively worsening on serial films.

Key Facts
- Often goes unrecognized with delay in diagnosis
- Penetrating or blunt trauma to cervical trachea or chest
- Clue: Progressive pneumothorax and subcutaneous emphysema despite chest tube drainage
- Radiography and CT – "fallen lung" sign
- Repair with surgery indicated in almost all cases
- Delay in diagnosis results in stricture

Imaging Findings
Chest Radiograph
- Persistent or progressive air leak despite chest tube drainage
  - Subcutaneous emphysema
  - Deep cervical emphysema
  - Pneumomediastinum
  - Pneumothorax (often tension)
- "Fallen lung" sign
  - Lung falls away from hilum
  - Supine position, falls posterior
  - Upright position, falls inferior
- Fractured ribs, clavicles, scapula, sternum non-specific
- Air surrounding the bronchus (ring around the bronchus sign)
- Endotracheal tube
  - Tip directed to right relative to the tracheal lumen
  - Distended cuff outside airway in tracheal rupture
  - Balloon migration toward tube tip
- Late finding after missed diagnosis
  - 10% have no abnormal finding
  - Bronchial stricture causes obstruction and atelectasis

Tracheobronchial Rupture

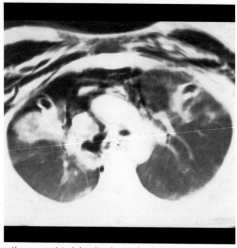

Right pneumothorax persisted despite chest tube drainage. Extensive subcutaneous and mediastinal air. Rupture right mainstem bronchus. Right lung has "fallen" posteriorly.

<u>CT Findings</u>
- 10% have no direct signs (tracheal defect or fractured cartilage)
- Herniated balloon of ET tube may have "Mickey Mouse" head or dumbbell shaped appearance (1 ear balloon, other trachea)
- Mediastinum shifted to side of rupture
- Trachea shifted to contralateral side
- "Fallen lung" sign
- Chronic: Stricture and narrowing

Differential Diagnosis
<u>Pneumomediastinum/Pneumothorax</u>
- May be seen due to contusion, positive pressure ventilation or esophageal tear (rare), bronchial tears also relatively rare
- Suspect bronchial tear if quantity of air progressively increases on subsequent films (despite chest tube placement)

Pathology
<u>General</u>
- Epidemiology
  - ○ Uncommon, in 3% of patients who die from trauma
  - ○ Delayed diagnosis common
    - ▪ 70% not identified first 24 hours
    - ▪ 40% diagnosis delayed more than 1 month
- Etiology-pathogenesis
  - ○ Direct compression between sternum and spine
  - ○ Sudden deceleration of lung with fixed trachea
  - ○ Forced expiration against closed glottis

Tracheobronchial Rupture

Gross Pathologic-Surgical Features
- From blunt trauma to cervical trachea
  - o Vertical tear at membranous portion of trachea
  - o From blunt trauma to chest
  - o Mainstem bronchi, most common, 80%
    - Tear < 2.5 cm below carina
    - Right side more common
  - o Intrathoracic trachea
    - Horizontal tear < 2 cm above carina

Clinical Issues
Presentation
- Respiratory distress
- Extensive subcutaneous emphysema in neck
- Diagnosis with bronchoscopy

Natural History
- Delayed diagnosis due to lack of specific signs
- Major airway tear should be suspected with progressive or persistent pneumothorax or pneumomediastinum
- Delay in diagnosis leads to
  - o Bronchostenosis and destruction of distal parenchyma
  - o Patient may require pneumonectomy

Treatment
- Must be repaired promptly with surgery in most cases

Prognosis
- Mortality, 20%

Selected References
1.   Mirvis SE et al: Imaging in acute thoracic trauma. Semin Roentgenol 27:184-210, 1992
2.   Unger JM et al: Tears of the trachea and main bronchi caused by blunt trauma: Radiologic findings. AJR 153:1175-80, 1989

PocketRadiologist™
Chest
Top 100 Diagnoses

PORTABLE ICU

Median Sternotomy

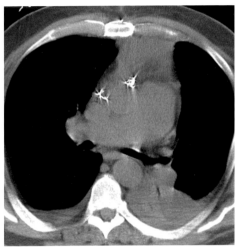

Retrosternal hematoma following median sternotomy. Hematomas following surgery are common. Progressive widening is an indication for re-operation. Small bilateral pleural effusions.

Key Facts
- Coronary bypass grafting is most frequently performed thoracic operation
- Mortality 1%, main complication rebleeding and mediastinitis
- CT is best to show complications of osteomyelitis, dehiscence, abscess and mediastinitis
- Mortality is up to 50% with complications

Imaging Findings
Chest Radiograph
- Immediate recovery room film, expected findings
  - Position of tubes and catheters
    - Mediastinal drains, chest tubes, Swan-Ganz catheter, endotracheal tube, nasogastric tube, epicardial pacing wires, infra-aortic balloon pump (if required)
  - Atelectasis in bases (90%) left > right due to:
    - Phrenic nerve cooling
    - Weight of heart
    - Difficult to suction left lower lobe bronchus
  - Edema, mild
    - Cardiopulmonary bypass "pump lung"
    - Anesthetic volume expansion
    - Intrinsic left ventricular dysfunction
- Mediastinal bleeding
  - Initial recovery room film baseline width
  - May normally slightly increase in width first 24 hours
- Sternal dehiscence
  - May be normal
  - Vertical sternotomy incision > 3 mm width
  - Wandering wires
  - Wire fracture incidental finding, not a finding of dehiscence

Median Sternotomy

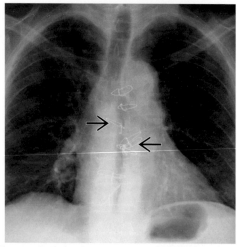

Sternal dehiscence. Vertical midsternal lucency is wider than 3 mm wires have pulled in both directions (arrows).

- Wires pull through sternum separating in either direction from midline

CT Findings
- CT best modality to show sternal irregularity, periosteal new bone, sclerosis, peristernal fluid collections/abscess, mediastinitis, retrosternal hematoma and edema
- Separate aortic dissection from rebleeding
- CT contrast sinography can show extent of mediastinal involvement of fistulous tracts

Nuclear Medicine Findings
- Bone scintigraphy and gallium scans can help to evaluate for osteomyelitis of the sternum
- Fracture of first rib may be noted with bone scintigraphy in patients who had median sternotomy and retraction during surgery

Differential Diagnosis
Aortic Dissection
- May also cause mediastinal widening in postoperative period
- Displaced intimal calcification

Pathology
General
- Epidemiology
  - Coronary artery bypass grafting most frequently performed thoracic operation, valve replacement #2
  - Incidence of complications is low (< 5%)
  - Major complications include dehiscence, mediastinitis, and osteomyelitis with mortality of approximately 50%

Median Sternotomy

Clinical Issues

<u>Presentation</u>
- Rebleeding
  - o Reexploration 2%
  - o General indications
    - ▪ > 1500 ml blood loss
    - ▪ Excessive mediastinal drainage
  - o Normal drainage:
    - ▪ < 300 ml/ 1st hour
    - ▪ < 250 ml /2nd hour
    - ▪ < 150 ml /3rd hour
  - o Evidence of acute tamponade
  - o In patients who rebleed, 20% picked up radiographically
- Dehiscence
  - o May be asymptomatic or nonspecific chest pain, cough, fever

<u>Natural History</u>
- Rebleeding occurs generally within first 24 hours
- Dehiscence or mediastinitis 10-14 days following operation

<u>Treatment</u>
- Rebleeding requires reoperation
- Drain fluid collections for mediastinitis
- Surgical debridement dehiscence, plastic surgery

Selected References
1. Templeton PA et al: CT evaluation of poststernotomy complications. AJR 159:45-50, 1992
2. Carter AR et al: Thoracic alterations after cardiac surgery. AJR 140:475-81, 1983

Thoracotomy and Complications

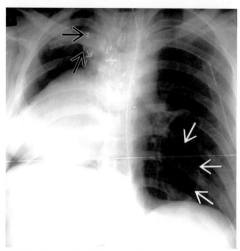

Cardiac herniation and volvulus following right pneumonectomy. The heart has herniated through the pericardial incision. The cardiac apex has rotated to the right. The normal pericardium is air-filled (white arrows). The superior mediastinum is widened from SVC obstruction (black arrows).

Key Facts
- Complications after lobectomy include atelectasis, pleural effusion, hemorrhage, air leak, infection
- Potentially fatal complications include pulmonary embolism, cardiac herniation, lobar torsion, pneumonia, ARDS, respiratory failure
- Normally, ipsilateral mediastinal shift after pneumonectomy
  - With contralateral or no mediastinal shift consider bronchopleural fistula, hemorrhage, empyema and recurrent tumor (late complication) in the post pneumonectomy space

Imaging Findings
Normal Appearance After Lobectomy
- Small amount of pleural fluid after the drains are pulled
- Effusion resolves during convalescence
  - Scattered lung opacities on side of surgery
Normal Appearance After Pneumonectomy
- 1/2 to 2/3 of hemithorax fills with fluid in 1 week
- Complete filling with fluid in 2–4 months
Normal Position of Mediastinum
- Ipsilateral shift to side of lobectomy
  - Returns to midline or close to midline as remaining lobes on surgical side hyperinflate
- Ipsilateral shift to side of pneumonectomy
  - Permanent shift
Complications of Lobectomy and Pneumonectomy
- Persistent pneumothorax, 10–20%
  - In supine patient air located anterior medial lower hemithorax (deep sulcus sign)
  - Upright and decubitus views will confirm, consider
    - Poor positioned chest tube

Thoracotomy and Complications

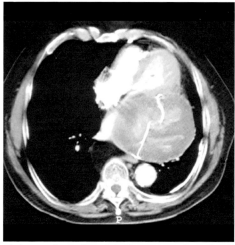

Retained surgical sponge (gossypiboma). Radio-opaque marker centered in the middle of the mass. Retained sponges often have bizarre appearances and may simulate abscess or recurrent tumor.

- Bronchopleural or bronchopleurocutaneous fistula - 2%
- Leak from suture line or bronchial stump: immediate post-op period due to ischemia or infection (late recurrent tumor)
- Esophagopleural fistula: Most within 6 weeks of surgery, may result from adenitis, empyema, recurrent tumor
- Bronchial stump dehiscence
  - Persistent pneumothorax
  - Failure to fill with pleural fluid
  - Drop in air-fluid level of > 2 cm
- Hydrothorax - excessive pleural fluid
  - Poorly positioned chest tube
  - Poorly positioned catheter with injection of fluid into pleura
  - Thoracic duct injury and chylothorax
- Hemothorax
  - From systemic, intercostals, mediastinal vessels laceration
  - Must be drained with chest tube or surgically ligate
  - Delay in treatment may result in fibrothorax and require decortication
- Empyema < 5%
  - Surgical contamination or from a bronchopleural fistula
  - Must be drained with chest tube
  - Delay in treatment may result in fibrothorax and require decortication
- Lung opacities nonspecific from atelectasis and edema common in immediate postoperative period
  - Pneumonia
    - Nosocomial, bronchopneumonia
    - Result of mechanical ventilation, narcotics, splinting, poor cough reflex, aspiration
  - Hematoma
    - Post-operative changes
    - Pulmonary hemorrhage resolves rapidly

Thoracotomy and Complications

- Pulmonary hematomas may persist for weeks
  - o Abnormal mediastinum: If no shift or contralateral shift of mediastinum away from pneumonectomy space
    - Consider bronchopleural fistula, hemorrhage, empyema, chylothorax, recurrent tumor (late complication)
  - o Elevated hemidiaphragm
    - Consider injury to phrenic nerve, atelectasis, pulmonary embolism or subphrenic abscess
- Cardiac herniation pericardial defect
  - o Following intrapericardial pneumonectomy, usually right pneumonectomy
  - o Circulatory collapse
  - o Right side – cardiac dextrorotation: Apex lies against right chest wall
    - "Snow cone" appearance
  - o Left side – cardiac levorotation
- Post pneumonectomy syndrome (delayed complication)
  - o After left pneumonectomy
    - Distal trachea and left main bronchus compressed between aorta and pulmonary artery
  - o After right pneumonectomy
    - Narrowed right upper lobe, bronchus intermedius and/or right middle lobe bronchi
    - Compressed between right pulmonary artery and spine
- Torsion of a lobe or lung
  - o After lobectomy
  - o Remaining lobe rotates on its bronchovascular pedicle
  - o 180-degree torsion leads to ischemia, infarction, gangrene
  - o Right upper lobectomy with torsion of right middle lobe (most common)
  - o Consider if abnormal position and orientation of pulmonary vessels and bronchi
- Herniation of lung through surgical defect in chest wall
  - o Accentuated by expiration
  - o Progressive separation of involved ribs with radiography or CT

Differential Diagnosis
- None

Pathology
- None

Clinical Issues
- Lobectomy
  - o Mortality 2%; morbidity up to 40%
- Pneumonectomy
  - o Mortality 6%; morbidity up to 60%

Selected References
1. Kim EA et al: Radiographic and CT Findings in Complications Following Pulmonary Resection. Radiographics 22(1):67-86, 2002
2. Bhalla M: Noncardiac thoracic surgical procedures. Definitions, indications, and postoperative radiology. Radiol Clin North Am 34(1):137-55, 1996
3. Gurney JW et al: Impending cardiac herniation: The snow cone sign. Radiology 161:653-5, 1986

Normal Tubes and Catheters

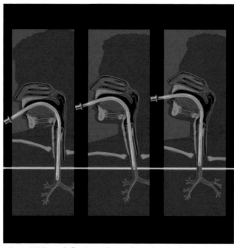

Intubated patient. With neck flexion - the endotracheal tube tip descends; with neck extension - it ascends.

Key Facts
- Radiography should always be done after insertion of a tube or line to assure correct position and identify complications
- Iatrogenic problems from malpositioned lines common and life-threatening

Imaging Findings
Endotracheal Tubes
- Normal ET tube tip should be 3 to 5 cm above carina
- Neutral head and neck
  - Tip of tube 5 to 7 cm from carina
- Cervical flexion
  - Tip of mandible overlies clavicles
  - ET tube may descend 2 cm
  - Tip is now 3 to 5 cm from carina
- Cervical extension
  - Tip of mandible off film
  - 2 cm ascent of tip
  - Tip is now 7 to 9 cm from carina
- Tube width
  - Ideally, at least 2/3 width of trachea
- Cuff
  - Should not bulge tracheal wall or narrow tube lumen
Nasogastric or Feeding Tubes
- Suction of fluid in supine position: Proper location fundus
- Suction of air in supine position: Proper location antrum
Tracheostomy Tubes
- For patients requiring long-term intubation
- Tip several cm above carina
- Tube should be 2/3 width of trachea

Normal Tubes and Catheters

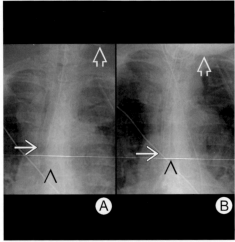

Normal excursion tube (ET) (white arrows). (A) Head is extended. Note position of jaw (open arrows). (B) Head is flexed. With flexion ET is now at carina (arrow heads).

Chest Tubes
- For pneumothorax in supine patient
  - Chest tube – place anterosuperior
- For hydrothorax in supine patient
  - Chest tube – place posteroinferior
- Empyema, hemothorax
  - Must be drained early
  - CT may help to plan drainage
  - Poor drainage will result in fibrothorax and require decortication

Central Venous Catheters
- To maintain optimal blood volume or long term drug administration
- Access from subclavian, internal jugular, antecubital, or femoral veins
- Ideal position, distal superior vena cava

Swan-Ganz Catheters
- To measure pulmonary capillary wedge pressure, reflects left atrial and left ventricular end-diastolic volume
- Access from subclavian, internal jugular, antecubital, or femoral veins
- Ideal position, right or left pulmonary artery

Intra-Aortic Counterpulsation Balloon
- To improve coronary artery perfusion and heart function (afterload reduction)
- Access from common femoral artery
- Long balloon (28 cm) inflates during diastole, deflates during systole
- Ideal position, tip distal to left subclavian artery

Surgically Implanted Catheters
- For long term venous access, usually for antibiotics or chemotherapy
- Reservoir in anterior chest wall soft tissues
- Catheter tip at distal superior vena cava

Normal Tubes and Catheters

Differential Diagnosis
• None

Pathology
• Polyurethane catheters are stiff for percutaneous insertion but will soften at body temperature, a correctly placed catheter may migrate distally with softening

Clinical Issues
• Interventional radiologists using fluoroscopy and sonography insert catheters more safely, faster, and better than physicians who rely on anatomic landmarks

Selected References
1. Tseng M et al: Radiologic placement of central venous catheters: rates of success and immediate complications in 3412 cases. Can Assoc Radiol J 52(6):379-84, 2001
2. Gayer G et al: CT diagnosis of malpositioned chest tubes. Br J Radiol 73(871):786-90 Review 2000

Abnormal Tubes and Catheters

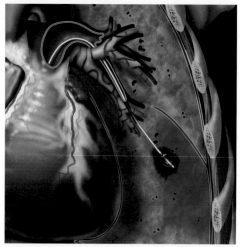

Tip of Swan Ganz catheter is too far out in a pulmonary artery sub-segmental branch. As the balloon is inflated there is injury of the vessel wall, pseudoaneurysm formation and pulmonary hemorrhage.

Key Facts
- Radiography should always be done after insertion of a tube or line to assure correct position and identify complications
- CT may be helpful when complications are suspected

Imaging Findings Complications
Endotracheal Tubes
- Malposition
  - Right mainstem bronchus intubation – atelectasis of left lung
  - Bronchus intermedius intubation – atelectasis of left lung and right upper lobe
  - 100% inspired oxygen, immediate atelectasis with bronchial occlusion
- Esophageal intubation
  - Dilated stomach
  - Poor lung volumes
- Vocal cord injury if tip is at level of larynx
- Sinusitis with nasotracheal intubation
- Barotrauma
  - Alveoli are overdistended and rupture from high peak pressures with mechanical ventilation
  - Interstitial emphysema
  - Air dissects along bronchovascular connective tissue to mediastinum
  - Pneumomediastinum and or pneumothorax
- Aspiration pneumonia
  - 5–10 ml of fluid may pool above ET cuff, deflation and aspiration may potentially develop into pneumonia
  - Suspect if normal air above cuff replaced with soft tissue density
Tracheostenosis (Late Complication)
- At stoma, tip or multiple foci
- At tip usually 1.5 cm below stoma

Abnormal Tubes and Catheters

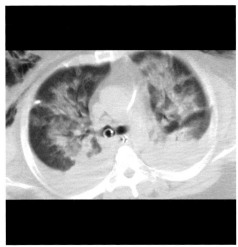

ET tube tip right mainstem. Other findings include diffuse pulmonary consolidation, small to moderate bilateral pleural effusions, and subcutaneous emphysema right chest wall.

- Circumferential, 1-4 cm long

Tracheomalacia (Late Complication)
- Extrathoracic, airway narrowing with inspiration
- Intrathoracic, airway narrowing with expiration

Tracheostomy Tubes
- Cuff in subcutaneous tissue, may cause tissue necrosis
- Overinflation of cuff or deflection of tip leads to tracheoesophageal fistula or into artery or vein producing hemorrhage

Nasogastric Tubes
- Bronchus, lung, or pleura
- Signs: Consolidation if fluid administered, atelectasis if occluding airway, pneumothorax if penetrate lung

Chest Tubes
- Poor position and inadequate drainage
  - Tube often in fissure, major or minor
- In the chest wall
  - Outer wall of chest tube is not visible
- In the lung resulting in bronchopleural fistula
- Sidehole in chest wall may lead to massive subcutaneous emphysema
- Tip impacting artery (i.e. subclavian) or esophagus may result in erosion

Central Venous Catheters
- Malposition
  - In subclavian, aorta or femoral artery
  - Through vein wall, into pleura or mediastinum
  - Into myocardium or pericardium
  - Into liver
  - Retrograde into a jugular vein
- Pneumothorax after placement
- Mediastinal hematoma after placement

Abnormal Tubes and Catheters

- Catheter breakage and embolization
- Aseptic or septic thrombus on catheter with pulmonary embolization
- Air embolism, rare but fatal in 1/3 of patients
- Infection
  - May occur early or late
- Fibrin sheath occlusion
- Thrombosis of vein
  - Directly related to duration of catheterization
  - Potential source for pulmonary emboli

Swan-Ganz Catheters
- Pulmonary infarction, from wedged catheter with or without clot, with or without inflated balloon tip
- Arrhythmias especially if tip in right ventricle
- Pulmonary artery pseudoaneurysm formation or rupture due to overdistention of cuff in small pulmonary artery
  - Pseudoaneurysm: Elliptical pulmonary nodule long axis paralleling vasculature within 2 cm of hila, usually right lung
- Pulmonary hemorrhage if aneurysm ruptures

Intra-Aortic Counterpulsation Balloon
- Too high, may occlude brachiocephalic arteries
- Too low, may occlude celiac, renal, superior mesenteric arteries
- Aortic dissection, balloon may tear intima
- Ischemia of lower extremity on side of insertion
- Helium gas embolus from rupture of the balloon

Surgically Implanted Catheters
- Infection, septic emboli
- Thrombosis, aseptic emboli
- Torn catheter between clavicle and first rib "osseous pinch"
- Rotation of pulse unit in the soft tissues by patient causing fracture or shortening of pacer lead (Twiddling sign)

Differential Diagnosis
- None

Pathology
- None

Clinical Issues
Treatment
- Infected catheter may clear with antibiotic treatment without removal
- Fibrin sheath-infuse tissue plasminogen activator, if unsuccessful exchange catheter
- Interventional snare retrieval for embolized catheter fragments
- Infection most common complication of central venous catheters, usually staphylococcus
- Fibrin sheath sign: Catheter may be flushed but not aspirated

Selected References
1. Tseng M, et al: Radiologic placement of central venous catheters: Rates of success and immediate complications in 3412 cases. Can Assoc Radiol J Dec;52 (6):379-84 2001
2. Gayer G, et al: CT diagnosis of malpositioned chest tubes. Br J Radiol. Jul; 73(871):786-90 2000. Review.

PocketRadiologist™
Chest
Top 100 Diagnoses

CHEST WALL

Elevated Diaphragm

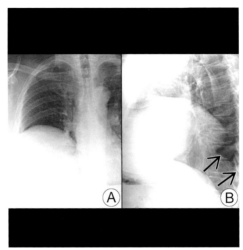

Marked elevation of hemidiaphragm on frontal views (A). Lateral view (B) the diaphragm returns to a more normal position posteriorly (arrows). Eventration and elevation.

Key Facts
- Elevation may be due to abnormalities in the diaphragmatic muscle, phrenic nerve, or adjacent lung, pleura, and abdomen
- Fluoroscopy can be used to assess for diaphragmatic motion
- Most common cause is eventration at right anteromedial diaphragm
- Most common cause for unilateral paralysis is lung cancer with phrenic nerve invasion
- Subpulmonic effusion often mimics an elevated diaphragm

Imaging Findings
General Features
- Best imaging clue: Fluoroscopy useful to determine motion
Chest Radiograph
- Elevated accentuated dome of diaphragm without meniscus sign.
- Costophrenic angles and posterior gutters are deepened, narrowed and sharpened
- Check prior films to determine chronicity
- Decubitus chest radiograph to assess for subpulmonic effusion
Fluoroscopic or Ultrasound Sniff Test to Assess for Paralysis/Paresis
- Diminished, absent or paradoxical motion – positive test
- Mediastinal swing to paralysed side during expiration
Barium Studies
- May show herniation of bowel indicating hernia or traumatic rupture
CT of Neck and Chest
- For mass invading the phrenic nerve or peridiaphragmatic pathology
- Thickened diaphragm muscle with traumatic rupture
MRI Findings
- Can best show anatomy of diaphragm with sagittal and coronal reconstructions

Elevated Diaphragm

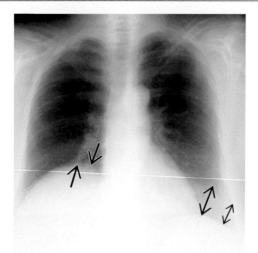

Paralyzed right hemidiaphragm. Double exposed radiograph at full inspiration and expiration. Normal excursion left hemidiaphragm (double headed arrows). Minimal excursion right hemidiaphragm (arrows).

<u>Imaging Recommendations</u>
- Fluoroscopy useful to determine motion

Differential Diagnosis
<u>Hernias</u>
- Foramen of Bochdalek (>75% left side)
- Morgagni (most on right, paracardiac)
- Traumatic rupture - 90%, left side
  - Contain bowel

<u>Atelectasis</u>
- Hilar displacement
- Juxtaphrenic peak (upper lobe)
- Mediastinal shift

<u>Infarct from Pulmonary Embolism</u>
- Splinting elevates diaphragm
- Humped-shaped area of consolidation

<u>Scoliosis</u>
- Elevation on concave side of scoliosis
- Spinal bone changes

<u>Subpulmonic Effusion</u>
- Simulates elevated diaphragm, dome shifted laterally
- Fluid may extend into fissures

Pathology
<u>General</u>
- Etiology Pathogenesis
  - Bilateral elevation
    - Neurologic due to cervical cord or brainstem injury, multiple sclerosis, myasthenia gravis

Elevated Diaphragm

- - Muscular: SLE myopathy or muscular dystrophy
  - Subphrenic due to ascites, abdominal mass, massive obesity, pregnancy
  - o Lung cancer most common cause of malignant nerve invasion
  - o Viral neuropathy usually involves right phrenic nerve

Clinical Issues
Presentation
- Usually no symptoms
- Bilateral paresis: Dyspnea, orthopnea, respiratory failure, hypercapnea

Treatment
- Usually none
- Diaphragmatic pacing in quadraplegia
- Long term results of pacing poor

Selected References
1. Shanmuganaathan K et al: Imaging of diaphragmatic injuries. J Thorac Imag 15 (2):104 – 11, 2000
2. Tarver RD et al: Imaging the diaphragm and its disorders. J Thorac Imag 4 (1):1 – 18, 1989

Empyema Necessitatis

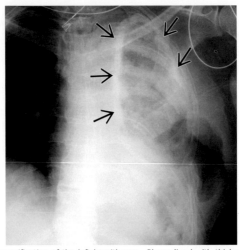

Complete opacification of the left hemithorax. Pleura lined with thick calcified rim (arrows). Irregular shaped air collection post-thoracentesis overlying lower left hemithorax extends beyond chest wall.

Key Facts
- Extension of pleural infection into the chest wall with or without rib destruction
- Most likely seen with tuberculosis, actinomycosis, invasive aspergillosis and mucormycosis
- Diagnosis with fine needle aspiration biopsy and microbiology
- Must be treated with antibiotics and usually drainage

Imaging Findings
<u>General Features</u>
- Best imaging clue: Loculated pleural fluid or mass with rib destruction
<u>Chest Radiograph</u>
- Loculated pleural fluid
- Soft-tissue mass chest wall
- Rib destruction and osteomyelitis
- Pneumothorax, loculated
<u>CT Findings</u>
- Loculated pleural fluid often admixed with air
- Extension into chest wall or ribs
<u>MR Findings</u>
- Also will show extent of chest wall involvement
<u>Ultrasound</u>
- Can be used as a guide for biopsy or drainage
<u>Imaging Recommendations</u>
- CT procedure of choice to demonstrate chest walls and rib involvement

Differential Diagnosis
<u>Tumors that Cross Fascial Planes</u>
- Lymphoma
- Lung cancer

Empyema Necessitatis

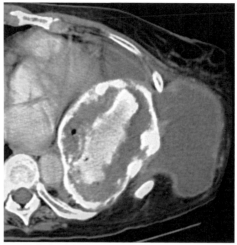

Complex mass with thick calcified rim. Pleural effusion. Fluid extends into the chest wall. Empyema Necessitatis originating from a dormant tuberculous empyema.

- Malignant mesothelioma
- Pleuropulmonary blastoma
- Primitive neuroectodermal tumor (Askin tumor)

Pathology
<u>General</u>
- Etiology pathogenesis
- Infection
  - Mycobacterium tuberculosis
    - Acid-fast bacterium
    - Chronic empyema may cross into chest wall causing subcutaneous abscesses
    - The collection may be enclosed by a thick calcified rind
    - Ribs often enlarge due to periostitis
  - Actinomycosis
    - Rod-shaped bacterium, anaerobe, sulfur granules
    - Oral colonization in patients with dental caries, poor oral hygiene
    - Aspiration, pleuropulmonary infection
    - Frequent involvement of chest wall and ribs
  - Nocardia
    - Weakly acid-fast bacterium
    - Infection more likely in immunosuppressed patients
    - May uncommonly traverse tissue planes
    - Must be treated because of potential for CNS involvement
  - Invasive aspergillosis
    - Dimorphic fungus
    - Mycelial form can invade vessels (angioinvasive) and adjacent tissue
    - Immunosuppressed patients e.g., leukemia, transplant recipients, AIDS

Empyema Necessitatis

- Inhaled
- Often fatal despite antibiotic treatment
  - ○ Mucormycosis
    - Fungus
    - Mycelial form can invade vessels (angioinvasive) and adjacent tissue
    - Radiology – same as invasive aspergillosis
    - Often fatal despite antibiotic treatment
  - ○ Blastomycosis
    - Fungus, yeast form in tissue
    - Rarely pleuropulmonary disease will progress to involve chest wall, and ribs
  - ○ Bacterial, nonspecified
    - Postoperative complication of thoracotomy, pneumonectomy or bypass surgery

Gross Pathologic-Surgical Features
- Pleura thin but difficult to traverse with either infections or tumor

Microscopic Features
- None

Clinical Issues

Presentation
- Fever, malaise, weight loss, chest pain
- Chest wall drainage
- Diagnosis with fine needle aspiration biopsy
- Specimens for smear and culture for aerobic and anaerobic bacteria, fungi, and cytology

Treatment
- Antibiotic treatment
- Tuberculosis, and some bacterial infections require chest tube drainage

Selected References
1. Winer-Muram HT et al: Thoracic complications of tuberculosis. J Thorac Imaging 5(2):46-63, 1990
2. Bhatt GM et al: CT demonstration of empyema necessitatis. J Comput Assist Tomogr 9(6):1108-9, 1985

Sickle Cell Disease

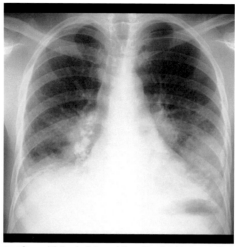

Multifocal areas of consolidation both lower lobes. Small right pleural effusion. Enlarged hila. Nonspecific findings in patient with sickle cell crisis. Note the absence of normal splenic impression on stomach bubble.

Key Facts
- Sickle cell due to abnormal hemoglobin which deforms when deoxygenated
- Acute chest syndrome common and recurrent, due to pneumonia or infarction
- Cardiomegaly common
- Bone infarctions cause classic H-shaped vertebrae
- Autosplenectomy: Susceptible to capsulated organisms like Streptococcus

Imaging Findings
<u>General Features</u>
- Best imaging clue: Expanded ribs and H-shaped vertebra, absent spleen
<u>Chest Radiograph</u>
- Lung
  - Lobar, segmental, subsegmental consolidation due to
    - Pneumonia or
    - Infarct
  - Interstitial thickening
    - Basilar peripheral lower lung zones
    - Sequelae multiple episodes acute chest syndrome
  - Heart
    - Cardiomegaly
    - Pulmonary venous hypertension
    - Pulmonary edema
    - Cor pulmonale
- Pleura
  - Effusions due to
    - Left heart failure
    - Pneumonia or infarcts

Sickle Cell Disease

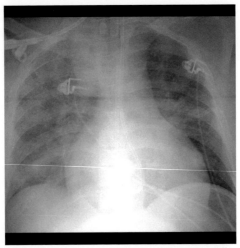

Fat embolism in sickle cell disease. Moderate cardiomegaly. Diffuse interstitial thickening. Focal opacity right upper lobe. Differential would include high output pulmonary edema or diffuse infection.

- Skeletal
  - Enlarged ribs (marrow expansion)
  - Bone sclerosis (bone infarcts)
  - H-shaped vertebrae (10%)
    - Step-off deformity superior and inferior endplates (Reynold's sign)
    - Due to microinfarcts
- Mediastinum
  - Posterior mediastinal mass due to
    - Extramedullary hematopoiesis
  - Subdiaphragmatic
    - Small spleen, may be calcified (autosplenectomy)

CT Findings
- Mosaic perfusion due to
  - Microvascular occlusion
- Acute chest syndrome sequelae
  - Parenchymal bands
  - Septal thickening
  - Peripheral wedge-shaped opacities
  - Architectural distortion
  - Traction bronchiectasis
- High osmolarity contrast contraindicated as they may enhance sickling

Differential Diagnosis
H-Shaped Vertebrae
- Gaucher's disease
  - Spleen not small (may be enlarged)
- Paroxysmal nocturnal hemoglobinuria
  - Spleen normal, no lung findings
- Alcoholics: No marrow expansion, spleen normal

Sickle Cell Disease

Pathology
<u>General</u>
- Red blood cells sickle when deoxygenated
- Genetic
  - Valine substitution for glutamic acid in hemoglobin (Hb S)
    - Normal hemoglobin (Hb A)
    - Hemoglobin S has some protection from malaria
  - Homozygous (Hb SS)
  - Sickle cell trait (Hb SA)
- Etiology pathogenesis
  - Acute chest syndrome
    - Multifactorial, exact cause rarely determined
    - Infarctions from thrombosis or fat embolus
    - Pneumonia
    - Upper lobe consolidation more likely pneumonia because oxygen tension highest in upper lung zones due to high V/Q ratio
- Epidemiology
  - 0.15% African-American population, 8% have sickle cell trait

<u>Gross Pathologic-Surgical Features</u>
- Microvascular obstruction by sickled cells leads to ischemia and infarction

Clinical Issues
<u>Presentation</u>
- Acute chest syndrome
  - 50% patients, common cause for hospitalization
  - New radiographic opacity with fever, chest pain, hypoxemia, and leukocytosis
  - Often recurrent
  - May be secondary to
    - Pulmonary infarction: From in situ thrombosis or fat embolus from bone infarcts
    - Pneumonia: Increased susceptibility due to lack of splenic function; classically encapsulated organisms (Streptococcus); Viral and mycoplasma pneumonia also increased
  - Leave residual scars which accumulate within the lungs
- Left ventricular dysfunction
  - High output failure from anemia
  - Renal failure (microinfarction of kidney)
- Pulmonary artery hypertension
  - Chronic vascular occlusion
  - Chronic hypoxia
  - Late in natural history of sickle cell disease

<u>Treatment</u>
- Oxygen and adequate hydration
- Pneumococcal vaccination
- Transfusions
- Antibiotics for presumed pneumonia

Selected References
1. Leong CS et al: Thoracic manifestations of sickle cell disease. J Thorac Imaging 13: 128-34, 1998
2. Aquino SL et al: Chronic pulmonary disorders in sickle cell disease: Findings at thin-section CT. Radiology 193:807-11, 1994

Pectus and Kyphoscoliosis

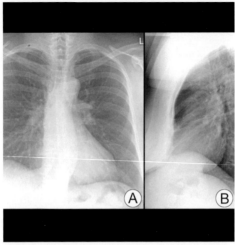

Pectus deformity. (A) right heart border is obscured and heart is shifted to the left. (B) sternum depressed posteriorly.

Key Facts
- Pectus excavatum may cause spurious cardiomegaly
- Pectus excavatum silhouettes right heart border
- Kyphoscoliosis may result from a variety of disease entities
- Severe deformity is associated with late development of pulmonary artery hypertension and respiratory failure

Imaging Findings
General Features
- Pectus excavatum
  - Right heart border is frequently obliterated because the depressed thoracic wall replaces aerated lung at the right heart border
  - Heart is displaced to the left and rotated (mitral configuration) may cause spurious cardiomegaly
  - Degree of depression best seen on lateral chest radiograph
  - In females, acute angle at medial superior margin of breasts
  - Severity of defect can be quantified by CT or MR
  - "Pectus index" = transverse diameter/AP diameter
  - Pectus index > 3.25 requires surgical correction
- Kyphoscoliosis
  - Usually convex to right
  - The chest radiograph is difficult to evaluate in severe cases because of rotation of the thorax and heart
  - Cobb angle
    - Lines drawn parallel to the upper border of the highest and the lower border of the lowest vertebral bodies of the curvature as seen on the AP radiograph of the spine, the angle is measured at the intersection point of lines drawn perpendicular to these
  - Neurofibromatosis I
    - 60% kyphoscoliosis, low thoracic short segment angular scoliosis

Pectus and Kyphoscoliosis

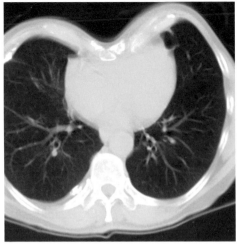

Marked pectus deformity distorts the heart. Note the calcified asbestosis plaques right hemithorax.

- Involves 5 vertebra or fewer in primary curve
- Scalloping vertebral body (posterior, lateral, or anterior)
- Hypoplastic or pressure remodeled pedicles
- Intervertebral foramen enlargement
- Transverse process hypoplasia
  o Lateral thoracic meningocele
    - Kyphoscoliosis, with meningocele on convex side
    - Round, well-defined, posterior mediastinal mass
    - Rib erosion and erosion of adjacent neural foramen
    - Associated with neurofibromatosis
    - Herniation of meninges through intervertebral foramen
    - Right > left
    - 10% multiple meningoceles
  o Ankylosing spondylitis
    - Kyphosis
    - Squared vertebral bodies
    - Ossification of costotransverse joints
    - Vertebral syndesmophytes, usually T9 to T12
    - Interspinous ossification
    - Manubriosternal joint erosion or fusions
  o Pulmonary artery hypertension with longstanding severe kyphoscoliosis

Differential Diagnosis
Right Middle Lobe Collapse
- Wedge-shaped opacity overlying heart lateral radiograph marginated by partially approximated minor and major fissure
- Sternum normal

Pectus and Kyphoscoliosis

<u>Large Right Epicardial Fat Pad</u>
- Sternum normal

Pathology
<u>General</u>
- Pectus excavatum: depression of the sternum so that anterior ribs protrude anteriorly more than sternum
- Congenital
  o Hemivertebra may lead to scoliosis
- Genetics
  o Associated with scoliosis: Friedrich's ataxia, Morquio's syndrome, Ehlers Danlos, Marfan's syndrome, muscular dystrophy, Neurofibromatosis Type I
- Epidemiology
  o Pectus excavatum: Frequently associated with Marfan's syndrome, Poland syndrome, scoliosis, and Pierre Robin syndrome
  o Scoliosis idiopathic in 80% of severe cases, female predominance 4:1

<u>Gross Pathologic-Surgical Features</u>
- Senile osteoporotic kyphosis: Compression fractures multiple vertebra and cortical thinning
- Pott's disease: acute kyphosis (gibbus deformity) at thoracolumbar junction, disk space preserved
- Infection spondylitis: Kyphosis, paraspinal mass, bone destruction, disk space loss

Clinical Issues
<u>Presentation</u>
- Pectus excavatum also known as "funnel chest" (the opposite anomaly – pectus carinatum is known as "pigeon breast")
- Most patients are symptom free
- Occasionally patients have cardiac (pulmonic murmur, mitral valve prolapse, syncope, Wolff-Parkinson-White syndrome) and respiratory (severe restriction) symptoms

<u>Kyphoscoliosis</u>
- Restrictive lung disease is the result of decreased compliance of both the lung and chest wall
- Restriction results in hypoventilation, hypoxic vasoconstriction, pulmonary artery hypertension, cor pulmonale, hypercapnia and respiratory failure

<u>Treatment</u>
- Surgical correction, if severe

Selected References
1.   Grissom LE et al: Thoracic deformities and the growing lung. Semin Roentgenol 33(2):199-208, 1998

The Ribs

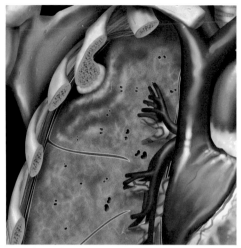

Osteochondroma of second rib may simulate a lung or pleural mass. This is the most common benign neoplasm of rib. Chondrosarcomatous degeneration may occur at the cartilagenous cap.

Key Facts
- Wide variety of rib abnormalities may be clue to underlying disorder
- Sensitivity of chest radiographs for rib fractures poor
- Most common benign rib tumor is osteochondroma
- Most common malignancy - rib metastases from lung or breast cancer

Imaging Findings
General Features
- Best imaging clue: Rib abnormalities easily overlooked

Chest Radiograph
- Calcification of rib cartilage
  - First rib cartilage is first to calcify
  - Men – calcification at margin
  - Women – calcification through center
- Congenital anomalies
  - Bony fusion and bifid or splayed anterior ribs (most common)
  - Ribbon ribs
    - Osteogenesis imperfecta and neurofibromatosis
  - Supernumerary ribs – uncommon
    - Cervical rib – 1.5% normal
    - Usually bilateral asymmetric
    - Can cause thoracic outlet syndrome
  - Intrathoracic rib
    - Arises in the bony thorax
    - Usually right side
    - From anterior rib or contiguous vertebral body
    - Extends inferolaterally to diaphragm
  - Omovertebral bones
    - Cervical rib articulating with scapula

The Ribs

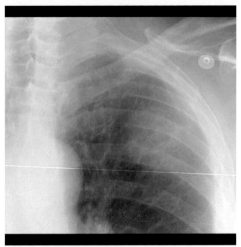

Mass centered over the anterior left 2nd rib. Margins are indistinct because the tumor is not in profile to the x-ray beam.

- Always associated with Sprengel's deformity – fixed elevation of scapula

Acquired Abnormalities
- Fractures
  - Sensitivity for acute rib fractures poor (20%)
  - Fractures of ribs 1-3 with evidence of mediastinal hematoma is likely to be associated with aortic or brachiocephalic artery injury
  - Fractures of ribs 10-12 consider liver, spleen and kidney injury
  - Flail chest, likely with fracture of 4 or more contiguous ribs
  - Abused children and alcoholics often have bilateral rib fractures at varying stages of healing
  - Cough fractures posterolateral lower ribs
  - Callus may be confused with lung nodules
- Rib notching
  - Inferior
    - Coarctation (most common): Ribs 3 to 9; lateral to costovertebral junction; from pulsating dilated intercostal arteries
    - Tetralogy of Fallot: Unilateral, usually left side
    - Blalock-Taussig shunt (unilateral right)
    - Neurofibromatosis
  - Superior
    - Quadriplegia, poliomyelitis, rheumatoid arthritis, scleroderma: Upper rib notching (ribs 3 to 9 posterolaterally)
- Osteomyelitis
  - Primary
    - Hematogenous spread: Staphylococcus aureus or fungal pathogen
  - Secondary spread from pleuropulmonary infection (See "Empyema Necessitatis"): Tuberculosis, actinomycosis, nocardia
- Non-neoplastic lesions

The Ribs

- o Fibrous dysplasia
  - Expanded rib with lucent or ground glass centrally
- o Tuberous sclerosis: Expanded dense rib(s)
- o Paget's disease
  - Bony enlargement, coarsened trabeculae, lytic and/or sclerotic
  - Starts at end of bone, flame-shaped edge
- o Langerhans cell histiocytosis
  - 2% with lung involvement, have rib involvement
  - Lytic lesions with no sclerotic margin and beveled edges
- o Brown tumor
  - Expansile lesion with lytic center
- o Unilateral rib enlargement
  - Reaction to chronic pleural disease, usually tuberculosis
- Rib tumors
  - o Primary benign
    - Osteochondroma (most common)
    - Enchondroma
    - Osteoblastoma
    - Neurofibroma, schwannoma: Rib erosion, notching, sclerosis
  - o Primary malignant
    - Chondrosarcoma (most common, in adult)
    - Ewing's sarcoma (most common, in child)
    - Fibrosarcoma
    - Primitive neuroectodermal tumor (Askin tumor)
  - o Secondary malignant
    - Metastases (most common): Lung, breast, prostate, renal, thyroid
    - Multiple myeloma

CT Findings
- Technique of choice for pleural and focal chest wall disease

Nuclear Medicine Bone Scan
- Can detect bone metastases before radiography (except multiple myeloma)
- Characteristic high uptake with Paget's disease

Differential Diagnosis
- None

Pathology
Gross Pathologic-Surgical Features
- Pathology easily missed due to
  - o Normally ribs poorly mineralized (less weight eases respiration)
  - o High kVp technique minimizes calcium
  - o No orthogonal views

Clinical
Treatment
- Rib fractures treated with analgesics, not splinting which leads to pneumonia and empyema

Selected References
1. Kurihara Y et al: The ribs: Anatomic and radiologic considerations. Radiographics 19(1):105-19, 1999
2. Kuhlman JE et al: CT and MR imaging evaluation of chest wall disorders. Radiographics 14(3):571-95, 1994

Index of Diagnoses

NOTES

NOTES

NOTES

NOTES

NOTES

NOTES